The
BUTTERFLY
Journal

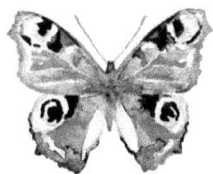

The BUTTERFLY Journal
facing cancer & finding wholeness

Halima

with a foreword by
Professor Robert Thomas, MD

ROSE GARDEN BOOKS
Glastonbury, England

Rose Garden Books
Glastonbury, BA6 9JQ, England

British Library Cataloguing-in-Publishing Data
A record is available from the British Library
ISBN 9780-9955103-8-8

DEDICATION

This account of my journey through cancer is for all those
going through similar journeys. There is hope, and we all have the
courage and faith within us to get us through. Believe in yourself.
Never give up – because if I can do it, so can you.

ACKNOWLEDGEMENTS

To Patricia and Teagan whose messages from beyond the material world convinced me to travel to Spain. To Rowan in Spain who kick-started my healing journey. To my children and my granddaughter, their support has meant more to me than they will ever know. To Dr. T, a family friend whose practical and medical advice helped me to make a very important decision. To all the amazing nursing staff at Musgrove Hospital, Taunton and Shepton Mallet Cottage Hospital whose never-ending kindness and support got me through hours of unpleasant treatment. To Gill, the very special MacMillan nurse who inspired me to write this book.
To all my friends who helped, and supported me, especially Caroline, and so importantly, all the love and guidance from beyond this world.
I thank you all so very much.

CONTENTS

PREFACE

The butterfly is a symbol for transformation, which is what I believe my journey through cancer has been. Looking back before my diagnosis I saw myself as a caterpillar, waiting to go into a chrysalis in preparation to emerge as a butterfly.

As the caterpillar, I was discontented with my life and had been for many years. I was sinking more and more into dissolution, despairing of ever finding my place in life. Somewhere in the world where I could feel I belonged, with people I could identify with and a purpose within a community. I was tired of being alone, both physically and emotionally. I was losing hope and something had to happen to bring changes into my life – and it did!

There are two reasons why I have chosen to share this account of my journey through cancer. Firstly, I want readers to be aware that there is so much we can do ourselves to support the amazing work of the medical teams who take us through our treatment, and secondly to prove that we are so much more than simply flesh and blood. There are other aspects of being human which although we might acknowledge them it seems we do not always include them when dealing with matters of our health. Although we are aware of our emotions and mental health we seem to disregard the energetic and mystical parts of ourselves. Many of us have a religion, or a spiritual practice that we follow yet when we are dealing with our health we generally keep these aspects of ourselves separate unless in desperation, when we might turn to prayer. Why do we, here in the West, acknowledge our religion or spiritual path, but not include them when considering our health and well being? We should not put all these different aspects of ourselves in compartments, but it appears we do.

The BUTTERFLY Journal

As a human being we have a physical body, an emotional body, a mental body and a soul (our spiritual body if you like). All these aspects are part of us and should be considered every day in every part of our lives. Any one of these aspects can go out of balance at any time and will need to be attended to not individually, but as a part of the whole. So It is essential to take all these aspects into consideration during any healing process in order to ensure a complete and holistic recovery. This means combining the amazing work of our medical scientists, pharmacists and medical staff with the age old natural healing remedies and gentler treatments offered by our complementary therapists of today, as well as visiting and familiarising ourselves with our inner worlds. This way we too are taking an active part in our own healing process.

It also brings us to the question: Is there an intangible life force at work in the world, helping, guiding and supporting us? Whether we believe this idea or not, it has been proven time and time again from people all over the world that some things in life are a mystery going far beyond any rational human understanding. Those who are religious might say this is God. Others might use the term Universal Energy, or guidance from 'spirit'. Our scientists would probably tell us it is simply an aspect of being human that has not yet been discovered. Whatever it is, it remains the one undeniable mystery for which humankind has been searching to understand since time immemorial. We need to acknowledge and incorporate all aspects of ourselves for true healing to occur: this is what my journey through cancer has shown me.

I live in Glastonbury, a unique little Somerset town in the South West of England. Glastonbury is renowned for its diversity, a meeting place for people of all social and cultural backgrounds, religious and spiritual paths and life styles. Generally it is a place where anything goes. Those who think they know me would probably say Glastonbury is the perfect place for me and yes about thirty years ago it probably would have been, but I felt I had long since outgrown what Glastonbury seems to be offering today. Before this journey I just felt displaced.

Glastonbury is also considered to be a sacred place. People from all over the world come here to experience the supposed sacred energies in the land and sample the natural healing spring waters. I have to be honest and admit I had never felt the sacredness that people here talk about. Perhaps I have never been in the right state of mind to be receptive. There are also many myths and legends associated with Glastonbury, e.g. the myths and legends of King Arthur for one and the legends of Joseph of Arimathea. All of these stories could be a book in its own right.

I moved here fourteen years ago under the guidance of my teacher Sheikh Nazim of the Naqshbandi Sufi Order. I had stepped out to follow in the footsteps of the Sufis almost twenty years ago, a new path taking me on an extraordinary journey, travelling both inwardly and outwardly. I feel it is important to point out here that although my own path is Sufism (how I came to this path is another story in itself), I respect all other spiritual paths. At the end of the day it doesn't matter which path we take to reach the destination we are all travelling towards. To me no path is better than another, but I can only give an account of my experience from a personal perspective. Perhaps I should elaborate here in case readers do not understand what Sufism is: it is the way of the heart, learning to listen to how our heart is guiding us. We can achieve this by developing our intuition. We are all intuitive, it is our sixth sense. It's just a question of understanding this and learning how to use it correctly. Sufism could be described as the mystical aspect of human nature and is therefore found in every religion and spiritual pathway. It is often thought to be only connected to Islam. This is because its cradle is in the Middle East and it's language is Arabic. In fact, it was here long before Islam. In Sufi tradition we use the 99 names of the creator, which are considered to be ninety nine aspects of human nature. All these aspects are within us. By reciting a particular name for whatever challenge we might be facing the light carried in the sound of the name causes a healing effect. I use the names like remedies.

But back to the journey. I had allowed challenging life movements to bring me to a full stop in my life – crossroads! Which way should I go? I dithered about, neglecting my spiritual practice. I was letting life in the material world get in the way sinking more and more into an unhappy state, not really understanding why or how this had happened. I was retreating into myself, but not in a helpful or constructive way. For the first time in my life I was beginning to understand anger, but I was not in a mental or emotional state to do anything about it. Looking back, I'm sure it was taken out of my hands.

It was late August 2018. On top of everything else a back problem from an old injury had been playing up and I had made an appointment to have a treatment I knew would help. After the treatment the practitioner, who was not my usual one, surprised me by telling me that the treatment might also have an effect on the lymph system.

Two days later whilst showering I felt a small pea sized lump in my right arm pit. Could the remark made by the therapist have been a warning? I left it a few days before I decided I had better have it checked out. A visit to my Health Centre assured me it was probably nothing to worry about and to leave it a couple of weeks to see if it disappeared. Two weeks later it was still there. I went back to the surgery and was consequently referred to Musgrove Hospital in Taunton for tests. The tests showed I had a tumour and it was not only cancerous, but aggressive too.

It was now October and I was due to go on holiday with my family. I felt numb with shock. I couldn't take it in. I don't smoke. I don't drink. I eat well and as far as I knew there was no history of cancer in the family. The rebel in me surfaced and I decided to go ahead with my holiday plans. It would give me time to seriously decide how I was going to deal with this bombshell. Part of me just wanted to shut it out. It must be a mistake, so for the next few days I simply got on with preparing for my holiday.

During those few days something strange happened. Two people independently and on separate occasions told me they thought I was living in the wrong country. Both felt I should be in Spain. Both also said there was a man there I needed to meet, and that is how my journey with cancer began.

The rest of my story is written from the diaries I kept to monitor my journey. The account takes readers through all the ups and downs of my journey, the anger and the fears, which made me challenge my own beliefs and my life in general. I have had to learn to put things in perspective, but it

PREFACE

also strengthened my faith in my own intuition and a belief in our creator. It illustrates how there are many ways by which we can help ourselves to heal from even the most debilitating disorders if our intention is sincere, our belief is strong and positive and we are prepared to work alongside the medical profession whose dedication never ceased to astound me. There are some truly very special people out there, from the understanding and kindness of the Red Cross drivers to the care and compassion of the nursing and medical staff.

I hope that by reading this account of my journey with cancer, readers might be inspired to approach their own journey in a fresh light.

FOREWORD

Halima, exceptional in many ways, is, I'm sure, similar to thousands of people who have had the trauma of cancer thrust upon them. There was an initial shock, a little anger and then a strong temptation to curl up under the duvet and let nature take its course. It was really helpful to talk things over, sitting down with Halima and her lovely daughter Liz, in her cosy home in Glastonbury. It was clear, with Halima's aggressive type of disease, that delaying medical treatments would have converted her disease from being potentially curable, albeit with intensive treatments, to incurable. She also had a type of cancer which 10 years ago had a poor prognosis but with the new generation of targeted biological treatments she was likely to do very well. These treatments have taken billions of pounds to develop by many thousands of dedicated scientists and fortunately we live in a country which can afford to use them despite their costs.

By the time we had finished two cups of tea she had stopped focusing on the negatives – how do I get to my appointments, I would be a burden to my friends and family, I would look dreadful etc. Instead, she started focusing on the positives – I can arm myself with new knowledge to reduce side effects, I can support others around me on the same treatments, I can help educate others following my path – which was the original inception of this book.

These new targeted treatments need a considerable amount of co-operation from those receiving them as they work by encouraging the persons own immunity to recognise and kill the cancer cells. Those with a better immunity, a better gut health, who ate more plant based phytochemicals and exercise regularly not only have better responses rates but less side effects.

The tipping point for Halima was when she realised that she had an active role in her management, she had not lost control of her destiny. True to form, she decided to empower herself with information to change her diet and lifestyle to give the treatments the best chance of working and ensuring her body and mind remained as strong as possible.

The changes Halima made, as well as the real life ups and downs of her personal journey, make fascinating reading. Her practical tips will help guide and motivate others during their cancer treatments. She highlights the importance of whole body and psychological wellbeing – subjects I fully endorse. I particularly loved the pictures she posts on Instagram such as the one using the essential oil based Polybalm to protect her nails with the quote, "The only patient on the chemo-suite with healthy nails."

This book is well written, entertaining and educational, expressed in an original format – I would strongly recommend reading this book after a diagnosis of cancer, as its advice will help, complement and enhance medical treatments.

Professor Robert Thomas Mb ChB MRCP MD FRCR

Consultant Oncologist, Bedford & Addenbrookes Cambridge University Hospitals; Professor of Lifestyle, Exercise and Biological scientist, University of Bedfordshire

Author of 'Keep Healthy After Cancer' (keep-healthy.com) Editor of the cancer lifestyle website: cancernet.co.uk

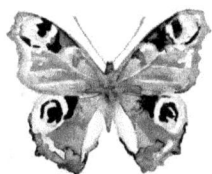

CASA DALIA, CADIZ, SPAIN
October 2018

I am here at Casa Dalia in Southern Spain staying at the house of my youngest daughter and her husband, trying to get over the numerous unpleasant hospital tests and coming to terms with what I am now facing, as well as seriously trying to decide how I am going to tackle this problem that has hit me like a hard punch. The news was delivered to me in a very matter of fact way, brutal to say the least. I left the hospital in complete shock. There was no consideration for the fact that we are much more than a physical body, but merely a machine that sometimes breaks down and needs to be repaired. I am angry, a rare emotion for me. I have realised I am angry with myself for allowing myself to be emotionally bullied by so many people in my life. Have I given myself cancer to sort this out? Am I going to go down the conventional route – chemo, surgery, and radiotherapy, or do I be a rebel and fight it by alternative means? I would like to think I have enough faith to go down an alternative route, but is this because going down the allopathic route I would be facing all my worst fears, and more importantly I would be going against my personal belief in energy medicine? I believe the human body is an amazing machine and with the right support can heal itself of anything.

This was proved to me over forty years ago when a 'freak accident' left me with a spinal injury which partially paralysed me for almost a year. I recovered solely by using energy medicine. These were McTimoney Chiropractic and Cranial Sacral therapies. I am not by any means suggesting there is no need for allopathic medicine, of course there is, but sometimes there are other ways too. Once I broke a small bone in my left foot. My foot was healed with herbs and prayers by a chance meeting with a man who happened to be a Sufi, something I knew little about at that time. He told me I would never have a problem with that foot again. I never have. Both these experiences changed my direction in life. Do I trust again, or do I conform and be conventional? That would be a new one for me. Cancer has so much fear around it. I am not sure in my present state of mind I have enough faith in my intuition to trust it. I wasn't in a good place in my life before this which has just added to my despair. I feel pathetic not being able to make my mind up. I have never been a ditherer. Anger is rising again. Is it just fear trying to bait me, tease me beat me into submission? I am going round and round in circles.

Dr. T is here, a friend of the family and an oncologist. Naturally as an oncologist he will recommend the allopathic route, but knowing a little of his work I know he also looks at support from natural remedies too. Dr. T had a chat with me explaining in detail the type of cancer I have. I had no idea there were different kinds. The hospital staff hadn't explained. They do their best, but their time is precious. Dr. T feels I should definitely take the medical route because my tumour is aggressive, but I could combine it with support from complementary medicine. I knew this would be his advice. The family want me to take this route too. I am still dithering, but I suspect this is fear speaking.

THURSDAY 25th October

When I arrived at Casa Dalia my daughter surprised me by telling me she wanted to introduce me to a man called Rowan who helped cancer patients with the use of diet and supplements. Was this the man my two friends in Glastonbury had mentioned? Was this why I had to be in Spain? I jumped at this opportunity, maybe I could deal with the problem this way. I could avoid chemo, and surgery. Meeting Rowan was one of the best things I have done, and he insisted on gifting me my session with him. I left his home, now describing my cancer as a bio-chemical malfunction not a disease and something that can be corrected. I came away with a list of supplements, reading material and hope, but I do still have that decision to make.

My children have been amazing, telling me they would be there to support me whatever I decide to do. I appreciate it must be difficult for them too, for a variety of reasons. None of us could take it in, but oddly we all felt the outcome would be good. My daughter said something else interesting. She felt sure I had cancer for an altogether different reason, which was to sort myself out. Inwardly I knew she was right, as I was feeling much the same and this is what I believe was the turning point. Now I have a reason for the cancer. I must concentrate on building a positive outlook. Dr. T had told me that it was those patients with a positive attitude who had the most successful results. However I knew I still have to make that decision. Which road do I take? or do I combine the two? My daughter has very kindly ordered and gifted me the supplements Rowan has advised me to take. Unfortunately most natural supplements cannot be acquired through the NHS, which is probably a reason why in general people take the medical route, but I see situations like this as prioritising and putting important matters first. The small initial pea sized lump in my arm pit has now grown to the size of a plum, which is frightening.

GLASTONBURY, ENGLAND
November 2018–May 2019

SUNDAY 4th November

The journey back was challenging. Our plane was diverted, so we finally arrived back in the UK at 3.30 in the morning. My journey back to Glastonbury was difficult too. This was due to traffic conditions, diversions, and the annual carnival vehicles slowing us down. I have sent off for the book on the diet Rowan suggested I should follow. Rowan has been in touch and we will speak tomorrow at 1pm. I still can't make a definite decision as which way to go, but inwardly I know what my decision will be. Thinking of the medical route makes me feel physically sick and I have had a fear of being put under anaesthetic. This is to do with an issue of trust. To put myself in the hands of someone I know nothing about who doesn't see things the way I do. Also all the drugs and all the poisons! Will my body at my age be able to withstand that amount of poison? I don't even keep any painkillers in the flat. I use natural remedies. I have stalled the hospital, delaying my appointments to give myself more time, but I can't keep doing this. In the meantime the book which Rowan recommended has arrived: The Plant Paradox, by Dr Stephan Gundry. The diet is brutal, basically mostly plants. Lots of green vegetables, avocados and lots of unsweetened coconut products, but I am determined to follow it. It feels right. Lots to think about and at least it will be less expensive, so there will be savings there.

MONDAY 5th November

I have an appointment at the hospital on Friday for an MRI scan. I will be facing one of my worst fears, as I am claustrophobic. My son will come with me. He too has been amazing, coming to appointments when he can. He works at the same hospital, as a psychiatric nurse. It makes such a difference having his support. I still can't believe this is happening to me.

THURSDAY 8th November – my grandson Reuben's birthday.

I am still undecided whether I am going to have conventional treatment. There is so much I am not happy about. We seem so far behind other countries in our approach to cancer – for example, my research has proved over and over again that tumours feed on sugar. This isn't mentioned at all. Surely one of the first things patients should be told is to cut sugar out of our diet. When I challenged the medics I was told, "but it's a comfort food!"

I understand the crisis our NHS system is facing, which is all the more reason for not taking that route. I keep thinking how our NHS seems to be like so much in life today which is that it too is fuelled by materialism. I must not let myself think this way, but my personal ethics do not want to support such a system. On the other hand the hospital staff are fantastic, everyone I have met has been so kind. They do their best, but like so much else in the world today they are trapped in a system ruled by greed, ego and ignorance, but their dedication amazes me. If I go down this road I will become a part of this unfair and seemingly egocentric money orientated society we have become. I believe and trust in nature and her wonderful medicine chest. In general, natural remedies do not have the unpleasant side effects that so many of our modern drugs have, and can be just as effective. Surely it is much healthier for us to avoid unpleasant side effects wherever possible. Ideally these two ways of helping us fight our health issues should work alongside each other. I think this is what I will attempt to do.

Oh dear, perhaps I am just angry because I may have to consider going against my personal beliefs and way of life. It's myself I should be angry with, for being too afraid to follow the courage of my own convictions. It's the fear factor rearing its ugly head again, and I don't have the energy to fight it and what would be the point anyway? But I truly believe I do have a point. I suppose I feel this way because I am of a generation when it seemed life was much simpler, safer and we were just happy with what we had. I could rant on, but I won't. I can't change the way modern society is developing in some areas, and I resent having little choice in the way I choose to live, because in some matters I have no option but to toe the line. Oh dear, time to go for a walk.

SATURDAY 10th November

The MRI wasn't as bad as I had thought. This was because I had to lie on my front and look down through a hole, a bit like being on a massage table. I questioned the dye that had to be injected into a vein, and was assured it was plant based and would cause no harm. I was advised to drink lots of water, which would then flush the dye out when I peed. I was given a choice of music to listen to while the machine banged and clattered away. Unfortunately the machine was so loud the music was drowned out. The whole session lasted 30 mins. What a relief when it was over.

THURSDAY 15th November

Today I am wallowing in self pity. I feel very alone, fearful and generally unwell. It could be the diet – I was warned of this, and assured it will pass. Also I am losing masses of weight. Starving the tumours, which I suppose can only be a good thing. I have no incentive to pull myself out of an impending gloom, a feeling of what's the point? I see no future. The children all have their own live and I am genuinely happy for them, but I feel so alone. I never imagined I would grow old alone. As I have got older I have lost the bravado to do things such as travelling. I seem to have lost confidence in so many ways. I have no self worth either, so why should anyone else value my life? It's my own fault of course. The only future I can see is so bleak I am not sure I want it, but I do know I want to see my grand children Reuben and Socie grow up, but I will not become a duty or burden to any of my children. Do I fight for my life? But for what kind of life? Where has my positivity gone? Perhaps its the diet. I understand it takes a while before I can expect to feel the benefits. There are certainly lots of emotions beginning to float to the surface, mostly anger, much of which although directed towards myself is also directed towards my ex-husband. This is a surprise. I thought I had moved on, but obviously not. I realise now I had allowed myself to be emotionally bullied by him. At the time I didn't see it. I just became more and more subservient: I was constantly trying to please because I wanted to be needed and loved, just like I was at the beginning of our journey together. I foolishly and truly believed we would be together for ever, grow old together, especially because of the way we met, our unique love story. He was the love of my life. It took me years to get over the way we parted. To me it was cruel and unfair. I am remembering how our marriage had been put under a great deal of strain, because we had been supporting various family members. I suppose eventually it broke us. I thought I had forgiven his behaviour, but it appears to have surfaced again. Unfinished business! Enough of this, after all I also had a part to play too, in that I had allowed myself to become so weak. I must stop writing and go out for a walk. Clear my head and get things in perspective. Today when we meet it's just like seeing an old friend. But that's on the surface; I realise there is a deeper level which is in need of attention and healing,

TUESDAY 19th November

I have felt very low these past few days, but today I feel much better. The reason being is that whilst meditating this morning and entering my inner world I think I was shown the reason why I feel so stuck. I am five years old, and its my birthday. I am sitting alone hiding in grass which is so overgrown it is higher than me. Tears are running down my face. I feel desolate, hurt and betrayed, and even worse I am powerless to do anything about my situation. I have been taken away from my grandparents, and the home I had lived in since I was born. Now I am in a strange place with two people I hardly know (my mother went to wherever my father was stationed during the war, whilst I stayed with my grandparents.) The war is over, my father is home and has taken a lecturing job at a college in Doncaster. The house he has bought is what I remember as the cream and green house because of its magnolia walls and dull green carpets, both of which I have had an aversion to ever since those childhood days. The house in Cusworth Lane is on the outskirts of the town, a lane leading to Cusworth village and it's a stately hall. It is pleasant, rural, but not a home to me.

It's strange, but whenever I have had to a face a challenging time in my life I have either dreamt, or sensed my grandparents around me. It is as if they are warning me of something I am going to have to deal with. I sensed them around at the beginning of this journey too. Those first five years of my life is the only time I have truly felt loved. Am I still stuck there? What can I do about it – is that why I was unable to save my marriage? I had given up because I thought – just like that five year old – that I was powerless to do anything about the situation. Is this a patten I have followed so many times in my life? Not this time. This revelation has given me just the kick up the backside I needed.

WEDNESDAY 20th November

When I found out about the cancer I decided I didn't want many people to know and so I have chosen to cut myself off from the crowd I usually hang out with. Glastonbury is a small town. Everyone seems to feel entitled to knowing everyone else's business. As a very private person I do not want to be the subject of gossip. One of the very few people who does know is my friend Caroline who is such a strength, phoning me every single morning to check how I'm doing. When I mentioned the child in the garden memory to Caroline she offered to help me go back to that time. We did this the other day through a visualisation exercise during which I was able to express my feelings to my parents and grandparents, explaining how I was feeling from my point of view. I also spoke to my five year old self. I explained we were now grown up and could do things for ourselves. I was also very surprised to realize my affinity with wild flowers must have begun at that early age. I sensed nature spirits. Even at that tender age I was becoming aware of the importance of nature and the floral world. To distract myself, and as an only child, I occupied myself drawing and painting fairies and flowers.

FRIDAY 23rd November

I've had a lengthy conversation with a friend who had been through the cancer journey and at the same hospital in Taunton where I was to be treated. She explained how she had found the treatment and the staff's attitude towards her. I found this very insightful and helpful. Rowan has sent me a link for a natural product which shrinks tumours, but it doesn't sit comfortably with me. I am up and down today and still indecisive about a treatment plan.

SUNDAY 25th November

Going for an ECG this morning. The last test before they want to start treatment. Decision time, no escape this time! During Caroline's morning call she told me she had come up with some insightful thoughts after reading the memoir I had written for my grandchildren. Caroline felt there was conflict going on between some different aspects of myself, describing these as the rebel, the saboteur and the victim. Thinking about her observations it makes sense and I immediately feel much better, much more in control. Caroline suggested I speak to these different aspects of myself – an inner council meeting to put it simply. The various life movements I had experienced had caused me to allow the saboteur with its sword of fear to quash the rebel who had been my strength, and so I became the victim, who expresses herself by becoming the pleaser. The following conversations are ones I had with these different aspects of myself, which incidently we all have within us.

REBEL "I am rebel, your strength and your power, your individuality and your uniqueness. I represent the potential of all that you can be in this life. I am the ultimate expression of you. In the folly of your youth you misused me, but now in your wisdom we can work together in harmony."

SABOTEUR "I am your test of expressing yourself, finding your place and purpose in the world. I test and make you question your belief in yourself and your faith, morals, and ethics. I wield my sword of fear and challenge you. I dare you to be you. If you let me, I will fill you with self doubt and fear, I am insidious. I creep into unexpected places in your mind, striking you with fear when you are weak then I can strike you with my sword of fear. Fear is my weapon. But I am not as powerful as Rebel who can make me shrink, tame me and then I will serve you well."

VICTIM " I am Victim, or at least I pretend to be because my twin,

Pleaser, needs to be satisfied. I can make you feel sorry for yourself when there really is no need giving Pleaser a platform to act from. This is because you have no idea how to work with Pleaser who only truly wants to work from unconditional love and not for any personal gratification. Wise up and try to come from unconditional love."

PLEASER "I want you to know me, to understand me, hear me, so I can please you so that you will respect me and notice me. I have so much love to share. I want to please you so that you will like me, love me, be with me. I am weak, and vulnerable. I will even turn my back on my friends, my family, my beliefs in order to please you. I have been working against you, not for you and so you became the victim."

I have found these inner dialogues with myself invaluable. I feel so much better, because now I understand. I know I can correct this. I feel positive again and have made my decision regarding how to get rid of the cancer. I must do whatever it takes to face and erase my fears.

TUESDAY 27th November

Still feeling positive and actually beginning to feel motivated. Thursday is D-Day. I must not let the saboteur unbalance the victim. I must stay strong. I have known in my heart all along what I was going to do. I just couldn't voice it. I expect this is because it would make it real. I am also surprised at how much I am beginning to enjoy my own company. I have ordered the book 'The Cancer Whisperer' by Sophie Sabbage. Sophie is a friend of the writing teacher I had when I wrote my memoir. Sophie's book is her story with cancer. I have made the decision to combine conventional treatment with energy medicine and diet. It is done and there is no going back.

THURSDAY 29th November

After seeing the oncologist I know I made the right decision. She gave me her views and comments on the type of cancer I have. Again delivering the information in a very direct and matter of a fact way, punctuated by fear. I notice cancer is very much dressed in fear, especially by the media. Shame on them. So much in life today seems to be negative and dark. I won't allow it to taint my journey. The oncologist wanted me to take part in a trial. She dangled a carrot, telling me that this trial would be ideal for the kind of cancer I had. I didn't take a bite. This felt wrong. I will check this out with Dr. T. I have and he agrees with me and told me his advice would be not to participate in a trial. I had told her I would give it some thought, and get back to her. Her parting words to me were: "Give us a year out of your life, it will be tough, and you can expect to be hospitalised at least twice." This only added more more fear and negativity into an already fear fuelled situation.

I suppose in all fairness to her she has to point out what could happen, but my issue is with the way these comments are delivered, just so matter of fact. I can't complain, she was pleasant enough. I suppose its all down to the individual delivering the information and the limited time they have as well as having to repeat themselves several time a day. I also have to accept that not everyone is as sensitive as me.

The children have all been great. One of my worst fears is being alone, but I woke this morning feeling that I am not alone. I can't find the words to describe how I feel, except I just feel different, calmer, more positive. Perhaps this is because finally I made a decision. I have done something I promised myself I would stop doing, which is to ask in my prayers to receive a rose to confirm I have made the right decision. This became a practice I have done ever since I prayed to St. Therese of Liseux many years ago. I had read in her notes when researching her life for the first edition of my book, 'The Way of the Rose', that she said she would manifest a rose to all those who prayed for her help as a sign that their prayers had been answered. It has worked for me every time, but I had began to rely on this too much and so I promised myself I would stop, which I did for many years until now. I have broken that promise, but I forgive myself because this is so important. I also realise my initial reasons for wanting to dismiss the allopathic route were the wrong ones and mostly based on fear, and my own beliefs, which I need to re-think. I will now wait to see if a rose appears in the next few days, which is usually what happens as a confirmation that a decision is correct.

My daughters want me to go to London after my first treatment, having chosen this route, but I feel to stay here. I am beginning to get a strong sense that this whole journey is about being tempered into the person I have the potential to become. Bring it on.

SATURDAY 1st December

Oh dear, the saboteur has struck and I couldn't get out of the way in time. I have come crashing down after reading the information pack I was given during my appointment. The side effects sound horrific. I can't see my body at my age being able to cope with the amount of 'poison' it will have to cope with. Have I made the right decision? Am I back to square one? But something very odd is happening. A very faint voice coming from somewhere deep within myself is saying "yes it can". I woke very early with these words swimming around my head, so I have got up, and made a cup of tea – very rare for me as I always start my day with hot water and lemon. I have come back to bed to write the following. "Its just fear rising again," the saboteur, don't let it in, but I am. If I don't make it, at least I will have tried. I really don't feel the cancer will kill me, but the poisons might.

I left a message with an association called Yes to Life the other day, but no one has got back to me yet. I just want some support. I want to talk with and meet people who understand, who have been where I am and have come out the other side. I am feeling so devoid of human understanding and company. I have prayed both inwardly and outwardly for the right support, but I know I have to be my own support. I am losing my faith, the footsteps I walk in on my path are disappearing fast, blown away by the wind of fear. That inner voice whispers again, "There is something bigger than a path, wider, it is a road." If only I could find it. Outside it's raining, dark, dull, cold and damp, not conditions conducive to raising the spirit.

MONDAY 2nd December

Well things aren't getting any better. I have had a message from my ex-husband to tell me he had just come round from surgery for bladder cancer! He also said he wasn't telling anyone apart from a mutual friend of ours, his present wife and myself. I felt sad for our daughter, with both her parents facing this at the same time. I told him he must tell her. I feel angry he has dropped this on me and that it was an unfair position to have put me in. I have also told him if his name comes up in any conversations I might have with our daughter regarding him and she asked me about him, I would not lie on his behalf. He must tell her, which he promised to do, except I have a feeling he won't.

A letter has come from the hospital: an appointment at 8.40 am. This is a difficult time for an appointment for me as I live so far away. I will call them as it doesn't say what the appointment is about. I suspect it is to see if I will take part in the trial and sign a consent form for treatment. I just want to get on with it now my mind's made up.

I have been for a walk in the Abbey grounds. I wandered over to the egg stone, a huge egg shaped stone by the Abbots kitchen which is thought by some to have the footprint of Jesus imprinted in it. It certainly does have what looks like a footprint in it, which forms a dent and which fills with water when it rains. Today to my surprise the little pool of water from the recent rain was filled with red rose petals. My sign? So my decision has been confirmed. I am definitely going to take the allopathic route. Finally I can voice it. I will journey down both allopathic, and alternative routes. The alternative will help lessen the side effects of the treatment, or that's the idea. I will also journey inward, through meditation, and prayer. I will return to my practice and I will use the light of each appropriate name of the 99 names to support each step of the healing process.

WEDNESDAY 5th December

Yesterday I had my second appointment and saw a different oncologist, a Mr. Graham, My appointed one was apparently away. This turned out to be a blessing. My son was able to come with me, and to cut a long story short it turned out that Dr. Graham knew our Dr. T, whom he offered to contact and which he did. Between them they came up with a treatment plan. Dr Graham phoned me personally that evening to tell me. I asked him if I could be his patient and he agreed. I feel so much better about it all. I have definitely surrendered to medical treatment, although I haven't signed any consent forms yet. I took Dr. Graham's advice and booked in for the flu jab too as it is winter and the flu season. I was told I could have a pneumonia jab too. I thought oh why not, they can be done at the same time. I have an appointment for these jabs later today. When I arrived for the appointment I was told I could only have the flu jab as they had run out of the other one. This turned out to be a blessing too, because if I had been given the pneumonia jab I wouldn't have been able to start my treatment as the vaccine was not compatible with my treatment drugs. My first treatment is scheduled for Dec 18th, with a pre-assessment appointment on the14th. Is some unseen force looking out for me?

I am feeling to have my hair cut in preparation for the inevitable loss of my hair, which will happen with the chemo. My eldest daughter sent me the following affirmation at 7.20 this morning: "I am physically, mentally and emotionally ready to enter a new phase in my life. I am ready to grow and get better." I am touched by her concern.

I noticed the charity shop opposite my flat has some really lovely new yarns, beautiful multicoloured balls of double knitting wool. I suspect one ball will make a pair of socks. I am going to buy some today and start knitting. I can make everyone socks for Xmas gifts and it will be a distraction from my treatment.

SUNDAY 9th December

Feeling pretty grim as I seem to have picked up a nasty cold, mostly in my head. I hope it won't interfere with my treatment next week. I just want to get on with it now I have finally made my decision. I have lost so much weight on the diet and still feel nauseous, but my mind set it changing. I feel clear headed despite the cold and more alive than I have felt in years and positive. After reading Sophie Sabbage's book I contacted an association called Yes to Life which she had mentioned in her book. I have been selective, using my intuition to source associations that might be supportive. This felt like one to contact. There is so much information out there it is like a minefield. This can be confusing and distracting, but this one felt right. I have had a phone call from a lady from Yes to Life. She was very helpful and caring, offering me a free counselling session. I have agreed, and a lady called Patricia will be calling me next Monday at 2.30 pm. Interesting!

I feel physically weak and I am running out of the supplements I have been taking. In spite of this mentally I feel good, but I do wish I could speak with others who have been in my position. I am hopeless on the computer, so joining any on line support groups is not an option and there are no support groups locally. So it looks like I am to go it alone. Maybe that's for the best.

My youngest daughter and husband flew off the West Indies yesterday. Her sister is holding the fort at No.10, their London home. I wish I could have helped her. They get back on the 17th or 18th and then they are off to the house in Spain for Xmas. They get back on the 5th Jan. Strange how I feel insecure when they are out of the country. I remember my mother feeling like this as she got older. I really do not want to become like that. I don't feel like painting or writing these days. I am just producing lots of pairs of socks.

FRIDAY 14th December

Pre-treatment talk today at 1.45pm. So it has begun. I feel surprisingly calm about it all. Even the prospect of death doesn't frighten me. It's the aloneness that is the worst. I have no husband or partner to be there for me. No one to share the events of the day with. Any day actually. I think back to past relationships. I always seem to be under valued, not respected, so I became subservient in order to please, and all because I didn't want to be alone. What a fool I have been and only myself to blame. It is as though I am being made to acknowledge all my past issues and deal with them now through this journey, so I should be grateful. I feel I have been given an opportunity. Sounds crazy, but this is how I am beginning to see this journey.

Can I heal myself? Oh dear I feel like a ball bouncing back and forth. I keep changing my mind so much, which is very unlike me. One day I am up, strong and positive the next I am dithering. Although I have to say generally positivity is out weighing the dithering. It's a real battle to change negative thoughts to positive ones, which really feels like a physical activity at times. The hardest issue for me is feeling that I am betraying my own trust in everything I have come to believe in through my life experiences. By surrendering to our NHS system of treating health issues,

I feel as though I am betraying myself. I have been such a staunch believer in natural healing methods.

This was proved to me when I had that accident in my thirties. But my trust in my intuition seems to have deserted me this time. Perhaps this is because of all the fear factor around cancer. I just don't know. I can't risk it. Or should I? Are my doubts because I am older and I don't have the bravado of my younger self? All these questions surface as I furiously knit socks. Knitting has become like a meditation a time when I slip into my inner world where all these questions bubble to the surface, ready to be explored, answered addressed and then wiped away. I realise the bottom line is about love. The only time I have felt truly loved was those formative years I spent with my grandparents, when I met my second husband and when my children were born. What a sad life!

It all comes back to that time on my fifth birthday sitting helpless in the garden of No. 48 Cusworth lane. Somehow I must get past this.

At the pre-treatment talk, which was given by a nurse, I was told I should avoid public places such as cafes, public transport and all places where people might be spreading germs. This is because the chemo will weaken my immune system. Great!!! I have get a thermometer, and if at any time I get any one of the long list of symptoms I am to ring the help line immediately. Then she launched into the various side effects I may experience. Not much to boost the confidence. I just wanted to run, forget the whole thing. I know they have to explain all the possibilities and they must be repeating themselves dozens of times a day, but it doesn't make it any easier. Personally I would have preferred not to know. I had to give a list of the supplements I am taking as apparently some may not be considered compatible with the treatment drugs. The nurse also felt my cold could be to do with the stress of it all, which isn't uncommon. She didn't seem to think it would interfere with treatment. I was advised not to eat yoghurt, soft cheeses, or shellfish. Not to use any beauty products that are perfumed. She also reiterated that I would probably be hospitalised at some time during my treatment. I left with a plastic wallet full of frightening information about the treatment.

SATURDAY 15th December

I have woken feeling very low. Outside it is grey and raining. Not a good time of the year to be dealing with this. The nurse I saw yesterday was the first one who I didn't feel comfortable with. In fact her attitude made me feel like walking out and turning my back on the whole thing. Talk about fear mongering not good for a sensitive soul like me. It is so scary now, but I am not going back on my decision. The good news is that the plum in my armpit seems to have shrunk. Sometimes I cant feel it at all! What is happening here? I haven't begun treatment yet so is the diet is responsible for the shrinkage? I have lost so much weight too, perhaps I am starving it away!

TUESDAY 18th December – D-Day!

I have just finished reading what I call a light distraction book, just a bit of fiction to take my mind off things. It was called The Bookshop on Rosemary Lane, by Ellen Berry. I mention this because it became a great source of inspiration, giving me an inkling of the inner strength I have. It's just buried under a lifetime of having no self worth. My cancer is in the breast. I associate the breast with mother, and mothering in every respect. I must learn to value myself as a woman, and a mother, and connect to the Divine feminine within myself. The Divine feminine is mentioned in my book The Way of the Rose, which I am currently rewriting. Fascinating it is all beginning to tie in together.

I left home at 7.30am (my friend Sky took me, and Caroline is to pick me up later). My appointment was for 9am. At 10.30 The nurse called me through to the treatment room. Rows of chairs hooked up to mobile machines. After six attempts by three different nurses to insert a cannula into my arm, the decision was made that I would have to have a PICC line put in my arm, which would stay there for the duration of the treatment, six cycles in all. By this time it was lunch time. Luckily I had brought a light lunch with me. I had to wait around until 4pm – the time I was told my treatment would be finished – and the time that was arranged for Caroline to collect me. I was told I must return tomorrow to firstly have the PICC line put in, and then the treatment. I was devastated and emotionally exhausted, I had been all geared up to get the treatment started today. We got home at 5.30pm. What a day, and tomorrow I have to do it all over again. I certainly feel as I am being tested. Do I really want to put myself through all this? It is so easy to get knocked off balance when I feel so vulnerable.

WEDNESDAY 19th December

Off we went again, another 7.30am start after a disturbed night's sleep. It wasn't as bad as I had feared having the PICC line put in. The treatment which I had been told would be six hours actually took seven hours because I had a reaction to one of the drugs. We left the hospital at 6.30 pm. I was exhausted and unsure of any side effects I might experience. Caroline dropped me off outside my flat. I closed the door feeling utterly alone I wanted to burst into tears, but I was too tired.

BOXING DAY, 26th December

It has taken me six days before I have been able to put pen to paper. I have just slept and dozed. On Xmas eve I developed a urine infection. I had to call the help line the hospital had given me. The receptionist didn't seem concerned, and told me to call the out of hours medical service, which I did. It was 7pm and I was told someone would be with me within the hour. I waited and waited, unable to sleep in case I wouldn't hear the door buzzer. I was exhausted, both emotionally and physically. At 1.30 in the morning a doctor came and gave me a course of antibiotics and told me if it hadn't cleared up in three days to see my GP. By the way, I forgot to mention that the laboratory had found no problems with the supplements I am taking – but I didn't give them all of them, like the CBD oil. The rebel had woken up.

Another upsetting issue to deal with is that I have to go to a little cottage hospital at Shepton Mallet, a nearby town to have the PICC line flushed. This has to be done every week. My first time will be on Friday at 12 noon. This means I won't be able to go away in between treatments. I will also have to find more help with transport. Another headache to sort out. However it's not all gloom. Yesterday I managed to go outside I walked up and down the garden path several times. I felt much better even though my legs felt like jelly, but I have to say that emotionally I feel stronger. I think the diet is working. I have a cup of hot water with ginger permanently by my side to help with the nausea.

Just before Xmas I had a lovely surprise. A parcel arrived from my two daughters. It was full of goodies to help with some of the side effects of chemo. Fantastic. There was a product called Quease Ease for the nausea, a roll up tube that you breathe in, all natural. A lovely rose scented moisturising balm for the soreness around my nose, due to the constant dripping, another side effect that wasn't mentioned. There was muscle balm for aching limbs, two pairs of lovely cashmere socks, matching beret, a pair of Ugg boots to keep my feet warm, some of Dr. T's natural nail balm and more. The Quease Ease is amazing. It works instantly. It has made me think, more people should know about these natural products. Perhaps I could put some gift boxes together. It would give me something useful to do as well as knitting socks, which I could include in the gift box. My mind is racing, a new project, just what I need ...

I had my phone appointment with a lovely lady from Yes to Life on Monday 17th which was very helpful. Just to have someone to talk to made such a huge difference. I also filled in a health questionnaire to help source supplements that could help my general health whilst undergoing treatment. A written report will come later in the post, containing lots of other helpful information. It sounds very helpful. There will be names of organisations too that might also be helpful. I am so glad I made that phone call to Yes to Life. Thank you Sophie Sabbage for your book.

SUNDAY 30th December

Farida, a Sufi friend, took me to Shepton last Friday to have the PICC line flushed. All went well. It is a lovely little hospital and all the staff I met were lovely too. I have had to see my GP as I still had the urine infection in spite of the antibiotics. The test was negative, although the result showed ketones in the urine sample. Apparently this was 99% due to the diet I am on. Too radical a change too soon, but not a big deal. I need to research the diet more and adapt it to suit my needs. Also I am not happy about losing so much weight, although I am beginning to feel in a really good place emotionally and mentally. I have decided not to be so strict with the diet and listen more to my body to tell me what it needs. Right now I am going to have a breakfast of porridge, followed by sourdough toast with under ripe banana. Yum. Although I have a horrid metallic taste in my mouth, so nothing tastes as it should. This is one of the main side effects of the chemo but it was never mentioned. Anyway the mere thought of food is mouth-watering enough and it's not for ever. Diet really has changed my mind set.

TUESDAY 1st January

Another year as 2019 arrives. It's very quiet here. I have been invited to Caroline's for lunchtime drinks and I am undecided whether to go, or not. I will decide nearer the time. It's only a small gathering, but I am concerned someone may have a cold. Also I am not sure what I will be able to eat. I have done more research regarding diet and a common consensus of opinion seems to be to listen to my body and let my intuition guide me as to what it needs. I have already introduced sourdough bread and I feel to add grapefruit. As I haven't felt like eating I think its important to have what my body tells me it wants when I do feel like eating, in keeping with my diet of course.

WEDNESDAY 2nd January

I went to Caroline's lunch party and really enjoyed myself. It was good to get out and do something normal. Another friend, Armena, called round in the afternoon. I was tired, but in good spirits by the end of the day. I had eaten and slept well. I heard Sophie Sabbage on Radio 4 talking about her journey with cancer and her book. The programme was about four women who had recently been through challenging life movements. Also I have had an email from Rowan wishing me a Happy New Year and some information about a new product that helps boost the immune system.

TUESDAY 15th January, London

Had the second treatment on the 9th. My youngest daughter came down and has brought me back to London. I managed to negotiate extending my PICC line flushing by a couple of days. She met me at the hospital and we saw the two ladies who specialise in wigs. They bring a selection onto the ward for patients to look at and try on. Luck was on our side because I tried one on and it was perfect. There was no need to try any others and, even better, it was trimmed to suit me there and then. The NHS give a grant towards the cost and my daughter and son in law gifted me the remainder. I left with new hair. Amazing – every one has been so supportive. I feel very blessed.

I am enjoying a lovely week with the girls and my grandchildren. However, I feel much worse after treatment this time. I have really bad stomach pains and nerve-end pains. These are sharp pains that suddenly hit any part of my body and bring nausea, which means I can't eat very much. I have lost just over a stone in weight since I went on the Keto diet that Rowan recommended.

One of the things we did during my visit was to shave my head. Everyone was there, my daughters and my grandchildren. We made it into a fun occasion, including a bottle of fizz. I had been dreading doing this, but actually it's fine. A relief in fact.

I had an email from a lady called Haley from the organisation Cancer Options. Yes to Life had contacted her. This was part of the follow-on after the consultation I had in December. It was a full report on my personal circumstance and so helpful explaining the impacts of some side effects which hadn't been explained by the hospital staff. It mentioned the nerve-end pains, which I hadn't understood and which had worried me. There were also details of various complementary therapies that I might find helpful, as well as diet and supplement advice. The diet suggested was an alkali one not dissimilar to the one I was on and of course, absolutely no sugar.

WEDNESDAY 16th January

Back to Glastonbury. We left London at 7.15am arrived at 10.30 am Liz had breakfast with me then headed straight back to London. I was tired and went to bed at 7.30 pm. On the way back we had chatted about the gift box idea. I will certainly do some research and give it some thought. It could be just what I need, as my knitting project is coming to an end because the charity shop has sold out of the lovely wool. I must have made at least a couple of dozen pairs. I have been gifting them to the various friends who have been helping me.

THURSDAY 31st January

Had treatment yesterday. I am halfway through Yippee! Also great news the last MRI Scan showed that the tumour is shrinking. I am certain it is due to a combination of the chemo, diet and my inner work. During my morning meditations I asked for a name (one of the 99 names) that I need to recite which is appropriate for the particular inner issue I am currently dealing with. Each time I recite a name I see in my mind the tumours, three in all. slowly shrinking. Now they look like small beads, or pearls. Each day the pearls are getting smaller. Sometimes when I am chanting a name I feel moved to tears and I see a pin point of light shining on the tumours. Extraordinary! I have previously mentioned the 99 names and how I use them like remedies, working hand in hand with my sincerity of intention. There is a medical doctor in America called Dr. Jaffe who uses the names like homeopathic remedies in his treatment of some of his patients. Apparently he is having some astounding results.

FRIDAY 1st February

Not feeling too good today. My granddaughter Leili has been staying with me, which was so lovely, but now I am alone again. I have indigestion, unusual for me, and I am tired having not slept so well.

SATURDAY 2nd February

Its 4.20am and I have woken with my head full of information. Many women of my generation today are being recalled to service. In preparation for this many of us are being put through some kind of transformation. Could it be that my transformation is through my journey with cancer? I truly believe this could be correct. The information that has come to me went on to explain how important it is to go inward in order to find and connect with the divine feminine within us, which must then be balanced with our lives and service in the material world. We are all in service all the time, even if we don't see it as such. A kind word to someone, a smile to a stranger, a good deed, these are all the small, but significant actions I consider to be our real work, our service. It stands to reason the longer we have lived the more wisdom we will have acquired through our life experiences. The younger generations often forget this, often dismissing us before considering we may actually be a valuable source of information and help. It's all about BALANCE, which ties in so well with the message of the rose. Accessing the divine feminine prepares the way to bringing about this balance, not only within our selves as individuals, but between us all.

MONDAY 4th February

Having a rough couple of days. The weather doesn't help. It is grey, cold and miserable. Never mind, it will pass. I feel nauseous too, stomach pains and generally sluggish. I just want to lie on the couch. This has been the worst cycle yet. I have no feeling in my finger tips, or my feet, and my legs feel like jelly. Exercise is becoming uncomfortable. It is exhausting just to walk up the High St. It's a week after treatment, so things should pick up again if the pattern is true to form. However my attitude is still positive.

WEDNESDAY 6th February

I couldn't face food last night. Feeling weak, and tired. I feel frustrated too because my mental attitude is still very positive and there is so much I want to do, but my body can't support me.

MONDAY 11th February

Been a rough few days, but now ten days after treatment I am beginning to feel better. Yesterday was the first day I felt vaguely normal. I have been out for a short walk and eaten both lunch and supper. I went to bed at 10 pm which is very late for me, but great. I slept right through till 6.20 am but had to rush to the loo with diarrhoea. Not pleasant. I think it was probably all the vegetables I ate after hardly eating for days. I have a slight headache too. All part of the course I suppose, but still feeling positive. I began painting again yesterday. The idea of the gift boxes is fading. I am not a business person, so being practical this would not be the project for me long term. I was pleased I could admit this to myself.

SUNDAY 17th February

Had a good couple of days, en fin.

THURSDAY 21st February

I had treatment yesterday. I took the manuscript of my book The Way of the Rose with me. Working on it during treatment was a great distraction. Time flew by.

It's 5.15am, and I am unable to sleep. I have got up, and made a cup of 'real' tea, very unusual for me, but so what. I had woken with the memory of an exercise I used to work with in my clinic days. It is going into the heart by visualising the heart as a mirrored room, choosing a mirror, and working with the image on the mirror that was preventing a client from seeing themselves. Deciding to do the exercise myself, I found myself in a walled garden. It was one I had visited many times before in my inner world. The sky was the ceiling. The walls were covered in mirrors. Every mirror had images of roses. The phrase 'the sky's the limit' came into my mind. I was standing bare footed on the earth, whilst I sensed my feet pushing down into the earth. My body became a thick stem, my arms branches, and my head a deep red rose. I thought of my book and the message of the rose representing the divine feminine. So is this what this journey is all about? Is this journey of transformation to unite me with the divine feminine within myself? From all my research about the message the rose brings to humankind, this makes sense. The two readings I have had recently, something I haven't done for over twenty, years both indicated that I am undergoing a transformation which will connect me to the wisdom of the divine feminine within myself. Interesting! So there I believe I have it, my work ahead when this transformation is complete. I feel elated. I now have a purpose, a mission and the idea of the gift boxes has definitely faded. I am going to pick up my research and finish rewriting my book, and I know exactly what I want the cover to be. The inner and outer journeys are working together. Hooray! It looks like my daughter's suspicion and my own intuitive sense that this journey with cancer is my way of being transformed in order to begin a new chapter of my life. Unless of course I am going mad! Ha ha.

SUNDAY 24th February

I am in London again and feeling rough after the last treatment, but I determined to override it. My head feels as if it is filled with cotton wool. I have a permanent horrid metallic taste in my mouth tainting everything I try to eat and I have jelly legs.

MONDAY 25th February

Yesterday was grim I have a very nasty taste in my mouth and I feel permanently sick, so I am not eating although I feel a little better today. I am hoping I will not have to have the last two cycles of chemo. I will know more after the next MRI scan on March 4th and assessment on the 12th. Had some fantastic news today. My daughter has booked us a trip to Marrakesh in May to celebrate our birthdays. My daughters and I all have birthdays within weeks of each other, I sense the trip may be significant.

TUESDAY 26th February

I still have horrid metallic taste in my mouth, nausea and dead finger tips and toes. In spite of this I am still feeling positive. The thought of a trip to Morocco keeps me going. I hope I will feel well enough to enjoy it and won't be a burden to the girls. I must start working on my confidence and not be intimidated by other people's behaviour, or views. Positivity!

SUNDAY 3ʳᵈ March

On Friday I was up three times with terrible bowel problems. I didn't eat all day yesterday, but oddly I don't feel so bad as I would have expected. My friend Rosita is visiting from Oxford. She has offered to come back soon to give me some Reiki, which is a type of healing. I have been feeling my body needed some vibrational medicine, maybe this will be it.

Only one episode last night and not as bad as Friday night. Strange it only happens at night. Times like this are very challenging for those of us who live alone. This has definitely been the worst cycle yet.

MONDAY 4ᵗʰ March

MRI this afternoon, I will be glad when its over. I am sensing that the physical aspect of the cancer is moving through to the emotional and energetic aspects within me. I seem to get moved to tears very easily. I have been working with the names and noticed the emotional response I am getting.

I am still working on the rewriting of my book, and am wondering if I should include a chapter on intuition? I am also sensing to start replacing the Keto diet with a simpler alkali one as the Keto diet is quite severe. It probably helped to shrink the tumours, by starving them, but now I sense something a little gentler is needed. My research tells me that tumours cannot thrive in an alkaline environment. Also I need to put a little weight back on. I shall start researching alkaline foods and adjust my diet.

TUESDAY 5ᵗʰ March

The MRI went well. My son came with me which was lovely. It really does make a difference and he will be able to come with me to the assessment next Tuesday. My bowel function and stomach are still not right, so I am having to be very careful what I eat. Consequently I have very little energy. I tried to clean the flat as I usually do on a Sunday morning and was completely wiped out. Even just going over the road to the shop does me in. Gone too are the days of my regular walk around the Abbey grounds. I really miss my walks.

WEDNESDAY 6th March

Beginning to feel like food again thank goodness, although my stomach still feels a bit dodgy. A friend, Margaret, has come round and given me some Reiki. The following is an account of what happened. As she began I had a vision of a large black bird – a raven. At first I was fearful, as Margaret has a strong energy, but I silently prayed and the fear went. The vision continued and I noticed a large gold ring on one of the raven's legs to which a thin gold rope was tied. The rope stretched into the distance, whilst the raven hovered over my head wings outstretched. I watched the rope float to the ground to where it was held by the figure of a woman in a pale blue dress which looked to me like someone from ancient times, possibly biblical. I also knew she was symbolic, and shown to me in this way so I can understand what she represents. I knew this to be the divine feminine represented by the goddess Sophia. I also knew this is the energy this transformation is connecting me to as shown in the recent readings that I have had.

The symbol of a raven is the same as all black birds, who are considered to bring messages from God. As well as this, the raven represents the archetype of the student. As I read about the symbolism one sentence stands out: "Whilst there is nothing wrong with acquiring a vast amount of knowledge it is important to put this knowledge into practice. The raven is asking you to share this knowledge with others." I thought of my book. The raven disappeared and in its place I watched two little blue tits. Blue and yellow are the colours of the teacher archetype. The message the blue tit brings is resourcefulness and its archetype is the innovator. The birds faded and I relaxed into receiving the healing. I sensed certain energy points in my body being what I can only describe as being activated in some way.

SATURDAY 9th March

I am feeling very excited as I truly have a strong sense that a lot of healing is going on in different aspects of my being. I sense I am being balanced. I have always been more inclined to resonate with the inner world. This journey with cancer is making me address the physical/ masculine aspect of life too. I suppose it had to be this brutal in order to get the message across. Well, it's working.

TUESDAY 12th March

Assessment today. I am trying not to feel apprehensive as to whether I have to have the last two cycles of chemo. My intuition tells me I don't need it and Dr. T felt four would probably be enough too. We will see. I am aware the medics go by the book so to speak.

Caroline showed me an article in the local Gazette about two ladies who are making up gift boxes for cancer patients. I emailed them offering to share the information I had collected. I am so glad someone is doing this. I don't feel so bad now about dropping the idea.

WEDNESDAY 13th March

Assessment went well. My son and I saw Dr. Graham who said It was up to me whether I completed the six cycles. I asked his opinion and told him what Dr. T had thought. Dr. Graham advised me to complete the treatment but with reduced doses of the chemo drugs. He advised this because I had had such a good result so far in that the tumours had shrunk, so it was worth completing six cycles as they could shrink even more. It made sense so I have agreed. I had had a feeling this would be his opinion. He also said it would make surgery easier. I explained I had a holiday planned and would like to go. I didn't say where I was going since when I had previously mentioned a trip to Morocco I was advised against it. It was agreed that I could have the surgery when I got back. Tomorrow I go for cycle five.

THURSDAY 14th March

Treatment went well and was all done by 3pm. I am not feeling too good though. The unpleasant taste is still a problem as everything tastes like shit. I have no energy and my head is fuzzy, but internally I feel positive and at peace.

Caroline lent me a book by Diane Cooper, which has inspired me and given me some information for the rewrite of my own book. I am still working with the 99 names.

SATURDAY 16th March

Not much to report, except I am writing furiously and enjoying the distraction, although I have to take lots of breaks to pace myself. All good.

MONDAY 18th March

Today I have woken with a head full of cotton wool, which makes concentration difficult.

Rosita came as arranged and gave me more Reiki, I can't say I felt anything physically, except I felt the need to breathe very deeply and widely, as if something was opening, or awakening, but I did have the following vision. I sensed a male presence or energy around me. I wondered if the healing was preparing me for the new energy Teagan had mentioned when reading the Runes. I felt as if something was being put into my hands. I sensed I had a garnet in my right hand and an emerald in my left. I also sensed a pair of swallows hovering around my left side. My head felt clearer. I must look up the symbolism of garnets and emeralds. I do know my birthstone is the emerald. Apparently, the swallow represents the archetype of recipient. Its message is acceptance, the last stage in what is said to be the five stages of healing following denial, anger, bargaining and depression. This makes sense to me.

Looking up the symbolism of garnet and emerald I found the following information: garnets are reputed to be stones of strength, higher thinking and self-empowerment. They are considered to be a deeply spiritual stone, inspiring contemplation and leading to truthfulness. They are also to do with our service to others and friendship.

Emeralds are thought to be to do with truth and love. The emerald is known as a healing gem in that it has a detoxifying effect on negativity, transforming it into positive emotional energy. Emeralds are an aid for any transformational process. They are said to be the jewel of royalty and holiness. Wearing an Emerald helps one to identify one's life purpose in relation to the universal plan. Emeralds are the birthstone for Geminis. All this is very interesting.

I had mentioned my woolly head to Caroline who thought this could be due to a misalignment in my neck, so I have left a message with my chiropractor Ann to make an appointment.

WEDNESDAY 20th March

I have woken expecting a phone call from Ann to say she could see me today. I got up and dressed early. Ann phoned but I was surprised to hear her say that the earliest she could see me is tomorrow at 11am. I had no choice but to agree. A few minutes later she phoned again to say her 9.30 appointment had just cancelled! I snatched a quick breakfast and was on my way. Caroline was right I needed a realignment. I am home again feeling much better. I hadn't been able to write when my head was fuzzy, because my eyes were affected. I have dozed most of the day and didn't want to eat but at 5pm I managed some scrambled eggs. I had been dreading the diarrhoea returning but so far so good. Went to bed at 9pm with every part of me aching. My fingernails are chipping and breaking off too. Perhaps this is because I have stopped using Dr. T's PolyBalm. Not sure why, I suppose I feel I don't need it. The numbness in my fingers and toes is getting worse. However I did have a phone call from my eldest daughter which was lovely. I felt much better.

SATURDAY 23rd March

Woke at 4.30am with an urge to do some inner work. I spoke to the cancer cells and as I did I felt a sensation in my armpit. In my mind's eye I saw my tumours again. This time they looked like tiny pearls. Three in the breast and what looked like a tiny string of pearls in my armpit. I spoke to them as if I was addressing a person. I told them I wasn't angry, and in a way I felt love for them. I asked them to give me an understanding of why they had become active. What are you trying to tell me?

The next thing that happened was that in my mind I was here in my garden, which has a Holy Thorn tree in it. The Holy Thorn tree is the famous tree connected to Glastonbury and the legend of Joseph of Arimathea when he allegedly visited Glastonbury after the crucifixion. Standing under the tree were two angels (the first I have ever really seen). One was dressed in green the other in dark purple red. I automatically turned my head to my right and saw a third figure dressed in saffron coming towards the other two. Then I must have fallen asleep.

The only other time I have ever seen anything I can describe as angelic was when my mother died. I had been sitting with her on that evening. My friend Lale was with me and I had never seen my mother so happy. She was sitting up in bed laughing and joking with us. She wasn't ill, just very old. She was ninety seven. At one point my eyes were drawn to the wall behind her where I was astounded to see two huge iridescent blue wings, one at each side of her. I composed myself and looked away. On the way home I asked Lale if she had noticed anything in the room. Lale said no, nothing visible but just an overwhelming feeling of love. Early the following morning I had a call from a paramedic to tell me my mother has passed away in her sleep. It wasn't a shock – I already knew.

Back to today when a few hours later I woke from a dream and a sense of a red light shining in my left side. I wonder why the light is red, because in Dr. Jaffe's work with the 99 names he talks about a white light. He explains that when the appropriate name is chanted with sincerity of intention the light from the name goes into the aspect of our being that is in need of healing. In the case of cancer, which Dr. Jaffe refers to as a disease of the soul, the light transmutes the cancer cells so can they return to where they should be. Repetition of the names peel away the layers of blocked energy from various life movements that had caused the cancer cells to become active. By understanding the life movement or attitude that caused this disorder the condition can be reversed.

I immediately recalled and understood a previous dream in which shadows from my past had been released. The dream showed me how I respond to people who treat me unkindly. I do not confront. I simply walk away taking the hurt with me which may have caused a blockage in my energy body, knowing it was their problem not mine. I would never stoop down to their level to argue pointlessly so I took the pain inflicted by the situation with me. I need to learn not to do this. Remembering my vision, I got up and went to look up information on angels. This is what I found: "The ladder of ascent to the first heaven, as recorded in the Koran, is held by two angels, one clothed in amethyst/red, the other in jasper green. Every believer will step on the ladder." A second reference I found told that when Jesus returns to earth – his second coming – he will be dressed in saffron garments. I can't put into words what I felt, except immense love and gratitude. I remembered the words from a poem my mother used to recite: "You are closer to God in a garden than anywhere else on earth...."

Today I made the decision to seek the advice of a herbalist who my friend Sarah is training with. Have decided against the three weekly injections of one of the chemo drugs Dr. Graham wanted me to take. I wanted to see if nature had a substitute and anything else I could take from nature's garden that would be beneficial. An appointment was made for May 3rd, her first available appointment.

Finally I can feel my strength returning. The worst effects of this cycle now seem to be over.

FRIDAY 29th March

I saw the surgeon yesterday, a Mr. Gill, who told me that I may not need a mastectomy. A lumpectomy would be his suggestion, which is what Dr. T had thought too. However in order to ascertain what to do I needed another biopsy, a scan and a mammogram. All this was done today. Not as bad an ordeal as I thought. Now I wait for the results.

I am continuing working with the names, so many are coming to me now, and I am watching the tumours which, from the small pearls had become tiny seeds, and are now dust, which I blew away. All that has remained is a miniscule thread under my right armpit just hanging there. When the doctor who performed the biopsy looked on the scan she told me she was uncertain what to do, because she couldn't see any sign of any tumours at all. She said all she could do was to insert markers in my breast and armpit where previous biopsies had shown the tumours to be. This is what she did. The procedure which I had braced myself for wasn't too bad.

TUESDAY 2nd April

Had pre-assessment today before last treatment tomorrow. The nurse dropped a bombshell. Apparently the results of a recent trial had just come through which suggested that after chemo, patients should then continue with more cycles of two of the chemo drugs for another six months. However because my last ECG had shown a slight decrease of 10% in my heart function, I should have a course of a drug called Ramapril to correct this, before putting me back on Herceptin, the drug that had caused it. Unbelievable. I told the nurse I didn't feel comfortable with this suggestion. She excused herself and left the room to confer with Dr. Graham. On return the nurse asked me if I would be prepared to have several months of three weekly injections instead after the course of Ramapril had done its job. I refused, because if I had this assessment two days earlier the trial results would have not come through and these suggestions would not have been offered. Makes me think!

WEDNESDAY 3rd April

Last treatment, YIPPEE! All good, I just hope the effects won't be too bad and I can recover enough to enjoy our trip to Marrakesh. After treatment I had the PICC line removed. I went home elated, and celebrated by buying a large potato and making some chips. I felt sad there was no one to share them with, but so happy I had made it, but I didn't particularly enjoy the chips.

I have made a start on the front cover of my book. So far so good.

SUNDAY 6th April

Its been a rough couple of days. The side effects kicked in early this time. Legs like jelly and a fuzzy head, which is affecting my balance, but I have managed to almost complete my book cover and I am happy with it. I have decided to go to London for Easter if I feel well enough, 20–24th April.

THURSDAY 11th April

I have had to cancel my two appointments for today as I feel too weak. This is definitely the worst I have been. I suppose it is the build up of all the poison in my body. I am completely drained of energy and can hardly move as my legs are like jelly. Migraines coming and going. I can't read or watch TV or use the computer. So boring!! I have being doing inner work on my inner child while in the garden, which I believe I have now released and at the same time I think I released my grandparents from their seeming compulsion to continue to look after look after my interests, even after death. All good. I now have an appointment with the surgeon for Thursday next.

FRIDAY 12th April

A better day than yesterday. I think I just needed to rest. I am not very good at doing nothing, and have probably overdone things. I must get stronger before surgery.

MONDAY 15th April

I can't believe how quickly time is passing. I walked to Morrison's yesterday and it almost did me in, but I made it. My legs are so weak and I am unsteady on them but I am determined to build up my strength. I also feel as I am about to go down with a head cold. The weather is unbelievably cold for April. This is not helpful. I need to seriously immerse myself in a project, not just think about it. Also I need to think seriously about building a life here in Glastonbury, making my peace with this enigmatic place. In so many ways it is the perfect place for me to do my kind of work, but there is also so much that is false and I can't find my place amongst it all. I am absolutely convinced that all the inner work I have being doing is almost certainly helping the cancer cells to disappear. I can still see the minute thread with two or three tiny 'seeds' on it just sort of hanging in my armpit. I did more inner work asking my ex-husband to let me go during this time and I had a sense of us finally saying goodbye. I am beginning to get a sense of a very new person emerging out of my old self. Never too late!

WEDNESDAY 17th April

Slowly beginning to feel better, although my legs are still numb, as are my fingertips. I woke with an image of a butterfly just beginning to emerge from its chrysalis. As I drew back the curtains I was astonished to see a peacock butterfly. I thought to myself that it had come out too early. I am feeling a bit stuck, everything feels at a standstill. I know it will pass, but I so want all this treatment to be over. Patience!

FRIDAY 19th April

I saw the surgeon yesterday, and apparently the biopsy showed the tumour has disappeared from one area in the breast and was benign in the other area, so no more cancer. However, he still recommended a mastectomy, not a lumpectomy as Dr. T had thought. He did say this was purely as a precaution. A date for surgery has been set for Monday May 20th. I can't decide what to do. Part of me thinks it's gone, so I don't need surgery. The other me thinks I have come this far, just finish it off. After all, the whole journey is making me face my worst fears, which can only make me stronger. They wanted me to decide there and then, and sign the consent form, but I couldn't. I asked to be given time to make my decision. I wasn't going to be bullied into making a decision before I have thoroughly thought it through. I know I was trying their patience but I stood my ground. After all, it's my life. Thank goodness I am changing and taking charge.

In the meantime I continue to work with the 99 names. Al Qawi blows away anything that is no longer necessary and Al Hamid gives the gift of purpose. I feel to contact Dr. T but I know what he will say. All I know is that I need to get as healthy as possible before I have any surgery, if that is to be my decision ... I came home and celebrated by treating myself to a hot cross bun, which I didn't actually enjoy. How sad was that?

FRIDAY 26th April

Went to London for Easter. I seem to have a head cold again, legs still very weak and the unpleasant metallic taste is still a pain. I saw Dr. T and told him about the test results. He again reiterated that in his opinion I needed a lumpectomy not a mastectomy, and again just as a precaution.

He said some people might prefer not to have surgery and take the risk that the cancer would not return. He said there would be no problem with the heart and surgery, or flying, but maybe it wasn't a good idea to go to Morocco just in case! More food for thought.

SATURDAY 27th April

Still feeling rough with the head cold. No sense of smell or taste and jelly legs. It's such a bore and so frustrating.

TUESDAY 1st May

Woke at 5am, and did lots of inner work using the names that came to me. I had a treatment with Ann today for my back and was delighted to learn my back was in quite good shape and thankfully only minor adjustments were needed.

MONDAY 7th May

I saw the herbalist on the 3rd and have remedies to help the heart return to normal, as well as other remedies to help with the transformation. I found the session very helpful and reassuring. I was back on the home ground of nature's healing remedies. I also left feeling I had got to the root course of why I had given myself cancer. It was all down to the lack of love in my life, going back to that five year old in the overgrown garden In Cusworth Lane. So I must learn to love and value myself. Working with the names regarding this issue I am astounded by the results. I think I should write about how I use the 99 names, what they are and what they represent. I started way back when my treatment began with Al Wakil – trust. This is the name Dr. Jaffe uses quite a lot in his work. I felt to use my intuition and ask in my prayers to be given an appropriate name as I moved through my treatment. After Al Wakil I moved on to Il Jalil. This name connects to our family and ancestors. As I began to recite this name I had a vision just like when I saw my tumours shrinking down to tiny seeds then disappear, apart from the minute thread, which I presume will be removed during surgery. The vision was of a white dove flying away with shadows taken from my maternal grandmother, my mother, my daughters and grand daughters. Then I watched as garlands of olive leaves were placed on all of our heads. The olive of course stands for peace. Later during the day I had a phone call from my eldest daughter and we had the conversation I have waited years to have. Unbelievable. I went on to recite Al Haqq which clears unfinished business from past relationships. Then Ya Fatah which opens hearts, and Al Hamid to find my purpose in life.

WEDNESDAY 9th May

I had a pre-assessment yesterday with the surgeon, and felt pressured into having surgery. I know it is the medical route and that I agreed to going down this road but it doesn't feel comfortable. I asked if I could have time to think about it, but was told they needed a decision there and then. I felt intimidated, under pressure, alone and it was scary. So many conflicting opinions. I am totally out of my comfort zone. None of them see things from my view point, so what is the point in even attempting to explain. I am like a fish out of water and came away feeling very low and emotionally drained.

Both my daughters called this evening, but I was too upset to speak to them, which I know they didn't understand. I went to bed early and exhausted. I slept on it all and have woken knowing that I will go ahead with the surgery. Where the decision has come from I don't know. But I do know it's the right one. Part of me feels I am betraying myself in that my decision goes against all my beliefs. Have I just let fear get the better of me – has the saboteur risen again? At 9am I phoned the breast care clinic and gave them my decision. I have no idea where the decision came from except I know it is the right one. I will have the surgery. I am putting it out of my mind for now and concentrating on our forthcoming trip to Morocco. Yippee!

During my quiet time this morning a thought came to mind. Many years ago as part of my training I attended several courses at The Arthur Findlay College for psychic development at Stanstead. Once all the students had arrived we were gathered together to be divided into groups according to what the tutors thought our particular gifts, e.g. clairaudience, mediumship, healing etc, might be and which tutor would be most suited to help each individual student's development. Whenever

THURSDAY 10th May

I went I was always one of those left till the end, as no one knew where to place me. One of the tutors Mavis Patel told me all she ever saw when I attended the college was an eight pointed star above my head. I have looked up the symbolism of the eight pointed star and have been amazed by the following information. The eight pointed star is the old symbol for Morocco. Evidence of this can be seen in the designs in the stone masonry and carpet designs. One Islamic legend tells how Solomon used the symbol of the eight pointed star to capture djinns which are mischievous spirits or the material counterparts of humans, the dark shadows hidden in human psyche. The eight pointed star became known as The Seal of Solomon or Khalim Solomon. The Essenes (an ancient sect to which some claim Jesus may have belonged) used this symbol which they had inscribed on the doors of their homes. Ibrahim lived in a city called Ur, where excavations found evidence of symbols of eight pointed stars, often in the form of eight petalled roses thought to be representative of the Seal of Solomon. Here is my association with Ishmael, and the Sufis. Eight is an important number to the Sufi mystics. Ernest Scott's research reveals that the number eight reveals the innermost secrets of humankind – perfection. Ian Alexander refers to the eight pointed star as the Sufi star, and the breath of compassion. More pieces of my own personal journey through this life are falling into place. My connection to Ishmael is irrelevant to this book, but it is detailed in The Way of the Rose.

THURSDAY 10th May

I ventured out yesterday and went to Cafe Sol, my favourite cafe in town. Tucked away from the bustle of the High Street, Cafe Sol is run by two of the nicest people I know. It has a lovely friendly atmosphere where everyone is made to feel welcome, and, as many people will tell you (including myself), the best coffee in town. It was so good to be out again. New beginnings. I feel I am getting back on track, balancing my inner and outer journeys by going through this transformation. A friend, Sarah, reminded me of something my teacher Sheikh Nazim once said: "We need to fly with both wings", an indication that we must balance our inner and outer paths through life. Travelling my two journeys through cancer, which is taking the medical route for the physical manifestation, balancing this with doing the inner work for my energetic counterpart, will give me the balance I need to heal, to become happy and healthy. Last night I slept through the night for the first time in ages.

SUNDAY 12th May

During my practice today I was chanting Il Wakil again. I saw through my heart two swans, one black and one white. Looking up the symbology of the swan I discovered they represented transformation, as do frogs, and butterflies. All indicating changes on some level of being. Next I chanted Al Jamil and I saw butterflies around everyone in my family including my mother and both my maternal and paternal grand parents, who of course have all passed. The butterflies seemed to flutter back down through history to bibical times when I saw an image of what I perceived to be Jesus. I then began chanting Al Fattah, the opener. The image of Jesus staying with me. Is this the Christ Light?

Today I am leaving for London, and then on to Morocco. I am feeling apprehensive as I feel weak after all the chemo, but I am excited.

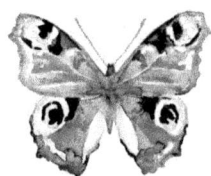

MARRAKESH, MOROCCO
May 2019

TUESDAY 14th MAY

We have made it, and here I am relaxing in the beautiful courtyard of our hotel. In spite of a disrupted nights sleep, as we had a very early flight. I feel great. It is very hot, but wonderful to be here in a country where I really feel my heart wants to be. The girls have gone off to explore and have lunch. I have opted for an omelette here in the seclusion of the hotel. England, Glastonbury and cancer seem so very far away. When we arrived I felt moved to tears to be back in Morocco.

Only Yesterday I was standing outside a shop on the Finchley Rd in London whilst waiting for my eldest daughter when a lady approached me and spoke to me. She told me she had seen me earlier and had wanted to speak to me then. She went on to tell me she had been stunned because she saw a bright light all around my head. It had stopped her in her tracks. She then told me I was beautiful. I was so shocked I simply said thank you. She was only a young woman and it occurred to me afterwards that maybe she was a being from another plane of existence. Who knows! but what a lovely way to start our adventure.

As I sit here in this beautiful peaceful place I notice how many eight pointed stars there are in the masonry around me. All those pieces of puzzle – Stanstead, Solomon, the Seal of the Prophet, Ishmael, Ur and Morocco are beginning to show me a picture and I am sure there will be many more pieces still to find before it is complete. It is all so exciting. It strengthens all my beliefs, giving me proof that we are so much more than a physical machine. Thank you God.

The BUTTERFLY Journal

WEDNESDAY 15th MAY

This morning I am once again sitting in my favourite little place in the courtyard. I have just completed my practice, and a thought has come to me. I am wondering if I should be considering spending whatever is left of my life in a country where people live their faith. It makes sense to me, my heart sings here, but can I be brave enough to 'jump'? We all slept really well and for me an astonishing thing has happened. My dead legs have returned to life. The heat doesn't seem to bother me either and I have so much energy. I feel I have been here forever. At 10.30am a guide my daughter has hired is coming to escort us on a shopping trip to the Medina. During our time with him, an elderly Moroccan man, I found a moment to speak to him about Sufis in Morocco and where I might find their communities I was surprised by his response. "If you are looking for Sufis you need to be in Andalucia in Southern Spain." This is where my daughter and son-in-law have their house.

THURSDAY 16th May

Yesterday I walked for six hours, apart from a stop for lunch, with no ill effect. I feel rejuvenated. I met a local man who told me all about the valley of the roses, which happened to be his home town, where the festival of the rose is held every April/ May. It is something I had hoped to go to this year. Cancer had put paid to that plan, but there is always another year. I also met an English lady who had lived in Marrakesh for years who told me that because of a convergence of ley lines in the square of the Medina there is a healing energy, and that many people visit just to hopefully feel the benefit of this energy. Interesting. So many plans are formulating in my mind. Our taxi is coming at 4.30 this afternoon. I feel sad to be leaving.

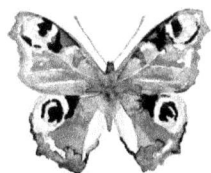

LONDON & GLASTONBURY, ENGLAND
May–August 2019

SATURDAY 18th May

Back in the UK after a challenging journey back, with traffic diversions and an extremely stoned, or drunk, taxi driver. We eventually made it back to the UK. Tomorrow my daughter is driving me back to Glastonbury. Surgery on Monday. She is staying with me until it's over. The plan is that she will stay until Tuesday morning and then my grand daughter will come on Tuesday evening and stay till the weekend. I feel so very blessed they are doing this for me. I am feeling remarkably calm. I thought I might have been nervous, but no. I am working with the names, preparing myself mentally and praying for courage. Having surgery is one of my greatest fears. So facing this is a big deal for me. It feels as if some invisible force has taken me over, and with it all my fears.

THURSDAY 23rd May

Well it's all over. I have to say I remained calm throughout. It all went smoothly, everything was on time. We had to be at the hospital at 7.30am so we left my flat at just gone 6am. I still can't believe how calm I felt. There must have been some magic at work. At 11am I was in a ward, sitting up and feeling great. All I remember is being taken to an anti room, to be anaesthetised, then waking up hearing some poor woman crying out. I remember telling the nurse who was with me that I needed to go and help the distraught woman. Eventually my daughter found me, I had been moved to a different ward. My son joined us too. The three of us laughed and chatted for about an hour before he had to get back to his department. Finally at about 5pm we were allowed to go home. I had been armed with pain killers and antibiotics which I did not want to take, but felt I should. The last thing I needed was an infection, so I took the pain relief for the first night, but resolved to manage without unless it became absolutely necessary, which it never did. I was also given an unbecoming pair of surgical stockings, or rather knee-highs, which apart from washing now and then had to be kept on for two weeks. Their only redeeming feature is that they are a rather nice greenish blue. They are very tight and uncomfortable especially as we are enjoying some very hot weather.

The worst part of it all is having a drain. It is a large plastic bottle which is attached to a cannula in my armpit. It fills up with excess fluid from the lymph nodes I am told this will be removed next week on my birthday. Great present! It restricts movement, especially when I want to venture out. Generally I am feeling very pleased with myself as I have faced my fears. Well done me. I have a follow up appointment on the 30th with Mr. Gill the surgeon, for the results of the surgery and presumably to see what delights they have planned for me next. One thing I have decided is no more drugs. I just want to recover and start creating a new life for myself. Now I need to build my confidence and find the courage to do so.

SATURDAY 26th May

I am feeling good apart from my chemo legs and finger tips. I am told that this feeling can last up to a year after treatment. The drain is very uncomfortable. I have to sleep propped up in case I pull it out in my sleep. Still, not long now.

I am also feeling, or rather not feeling, my right upper arm. The whole of the surgery site is numb apart from the occasional sharp pain searing through where my breast would have been, in my armpit and upper arm. I understand this to be to do with the nerve endings. These sharp pains, a bit like a pin or needle sticking in to me can be felt anywhere in the body without warning. The drain is becoming alarmingly full. I was given a replacement bottle which I was told I would have to change myself. The reason given for this was because apparently no one at either my surgery or local hospital were qualified to do it for me. I thought this odd as surely anyone connected with a medical practice would have been better than someone like myself with no knowledge of these things whatsoever. Red tape!

Caroline came round for moral support and as far as I know we followed all the instructions. What we hadn't foreseen was that I had been given a replacement bottle with a faulty connection to the drain. Consequently very little fluid was getting through. I was delighted. In my ignorance I assumed there was no more fluid to drain away, although the whole area was hard and swollen, but I wasn't worried and it was only two days to go before it was going to be removed.

TUESDAY 28th May

My birthday today, I can't believe how old I am – where have all the years gone? Yesterday I wandered along the High St, drain bottle suitably protected and hidden in a shoulder bag, when I noticed a row of prints of different places in Morocco in a charity shop. I chose one as a birthday gift to myself. I needed a bit of good cheer, as I am just beginning to feel the effects of the trauma of it all. I realised this after I had had a plea for help from a family member. I just couldn't deal with it and had to retreat into my own little world. I think I must have used my last bit of energy for the operation. I now need to get strong again and not let the needs of others hinder my recovery.

WEDNESDAY 29th May

The drain was removed yesterday, not a bad procedure at all. I felt elated and relived I have woken early. It is wonderful not to have the drain to contend with. Freedom. I feel my energy returning, but still need my own space to be quiet in. I would love nothing more than to have a few days just lying in the sun by the sea. Dream on. My finger tips and feet continue to have no feeling. I don't have much pain but I do have a soreness and sometimes a stinging sensation where the breast tissue, and lymph nodes have been removed. I will mention this tomorrow when I see Mr. Gill. I am also very tired most of the time and I am just spending the day lying on the sofa. Time is the essence of healing, so I guess I just need to be patient. My hair is beginning to grow, covering my scalp with a grey and white fuzz, not at all attractive.

Interesting that no one from the red cross has phoned yet for my pick up tomorrow, which is unusual. I will have to contact them as soon as the office opens in the morning. Bother. Generally I am slowly feeling stronger and beginning to make plans for my future. I have been continuing with my rewriting, and The way of the Rose is progressing nicely.

Examining the white fuzz this morning I noticed my eyebrows and eye lashes were growing back too. I will not have to look like an alien for much longer. I have been taking Kelp as a supplement to help with hair regrowth. It's working – hooray!

THURSDAY 30ᵗʰ May

I phoned the Red Cross and was assured that someone would probably call me this morning. My appointment is for 2.40pm. At 1.20pm no one had called so I phoned the Red Cross again as it takes an hour to get to the hospital. I used my mobile just in case a driver called at the same time. In my mind I just felt I would not be going to the appointment. The Red Cross receptionist was very apologetic and couldn't understand what had gone wrong. I was definitely booked in. Just as we were trying to find a solution my land line rang. I picked it up, asking the receptionist to hang on in case it was a driver. It was the hospital apologising for the lateness of the call but telling me they would have to cancel my appointment as the results from the lab weren't back yet due to it having been a bank holiday last weekend! A new appointment was arranged for the following Thursday at 4.20 pm. I relayed all this to the Red Cross receptionist on my mobile. She was immediately able to book my transport for the following Thursday, June 6th. So what happened there? All this just makes me feel some other energetic force is at work here. Who knows? I now have to wait another week for the results. Strangely this doesn't bother me. In fact I feel completely laid back about it all. I know what I was shown through my heart, and I trust without any doubt it is correct. Stockings come off next Monday. Hooray!

MONDAY 3ʳᵈ June – my youngest daughter's birthday

I have woken feeling a little down. Although there is little pain apart from the odd sting in my right breast, or rather where my breast had been, which is swollen with fluid. The underside of my right arm at the top is both sore and numb an odd feeling. This is what is bringing me down as I thought I would have been feeling better by now. I showered yesterday which was fantastic, but the dressing where the breast had been removed stayed put, although I was able to removed the drain dressing and all was as it should be. Maybe I should exercise more? I was given some arm exercises to do. I must make a start. I am beginning to think about what to do with the rest of my life. I had planned to go to the Margaret chapel for zikhr (a Sufi gathering when we get together to recite the 99 names, with music and prayer in remembrance of God), but it rained and I got engrossed in a film on TV. However it did make me think about why I had felt I had wanted to go to the zikhr. I questioned as to whether it was because I need social contact with like minded people? I am feeling very isolated. Shar, an old friend, came round yesterday morning and we enjoyed a good conversation. I need social interaction, but not with the nonsense of the cafe crowd, which used to be a social outlet. I feel the need for new social interests which suits me better at this time of my life, and to start getting out and about again, to find another layer of Glastonbury. I feel as if I am standing at the gate of nothingness and no-oneness. If that makes any sense? Oh dear! I had better get a grip.

THURSDAY 6th June

The melancholy has lifted, thank goodness. It had descended out of nowhere like a dark mist. I prayed for a name to help lift this and Ya Wakil – trust – came to me. After reciting this I bit the bullet and phoned the breast care centre about the fluid situation. They could see me at midday. Then I phoned my friend Sky to see if he would take me, luckily he could and so I was back at the breast clinic where a lovely nurse called Jane drained off another 500 mils of fluid. I felt so much better in spite of the pain afterwards. The drainage itself wasn't too bad. I am so glad I made that call. At one point Jane looked at me and said, "I shouldn't really be telling you this, but you have waited long enough, what with the bank holiday disrupting everything, but your results from surgery are back from the lab and it's excellent news." Even though I knew in my heart all would be well I was still choked to hear her words. Later today I have a meeting with Mr. Gill the surgeon. I am interested to see what he has to say and what delights they propose to do next. Mr. Gill greeted me with a smile, as he imparted the good news. He explained that the tumour in the breast tissue was benign and all they found was a tiny thread of cancer cells about two millimetres long, hanging from a lymph node. Inwardly I was quietly smiling. This thread was removed as was the node and as a precaution three surrounding lymph nodes. So it would seem a mastectomy hadn't been necessary. Dr. T had been correct in his opinion. Too late my breast has gone, but that's the way the NHS works. I was told it was all done as a precaution. Fair enough, I had consented to go down this road and I don't regret my decision. Another lovely nurse Lisa examined my breast area and told me all was healing well. Then she surprised me by saying "but you knew didn't you?" I just shrugged and grinned. She also said if any more fluid collected she would prefer it was left to drain away of its own accord. This concerned me as I could tell more fluid was already beginning to build up again. I will ask my herbalist if there is anything I can take to relieve this and also I will look into my inner world to see what I am still holding on to, as fluid can indicate holding on to old emotional pattens

Mr. Gill told me again that again purely as a precaution he recommends fifteen days of radiotherapy. I need to seriously consider this. It has just occurred to me that all those years working in clinics helping others, I am now having to do this same work for myself! Interesting. I feel such a dummy, why had this only just dawned on me?

I have begun work on my book about this journey with cancer. I am calling it 'Butterfly', because the butterfly is a symbol for transformation, which I believe is what this journey is about.

SATURDAY 8th June

Thoughts: The public's health should not be compromised by the greed to make money. For example, unnecessary drugs being prescribed when there is often equally effective, natural and less costly ways to support our health, and without the side effects many drugs cause. Thank goodness some GPs are now beginning to recognise this.

MONDAY 10th June

Disappointed I had to phone the breast clinic again, as I have have filled up with fluid once more and I know it will need to be drained off again. I am told this is not uncommon.

I have bought my ticket for London and hope I will be able to go. I feel a bit gloomy today, but I am going to the cafe. I have come home feeling much better for some social time. I have spent far too much time alone.

The first draft of my book 'The Way of the Rose' is complete, and I have taken the memory stick to Paul at Blue Cedar to print me out a hard copy. Exciting!

TUESDAY 11th June

I have been out and about again today and it feels really good, although I have to say I feel self conscious in my wig. Amazingly most people seem to think I have just had a new hair do, to which my response is 'I have just been to London'. A thought came that maybe I could make an audio version of my book and do it for charity. Am I getting carried away again? Hospital tomorrow for more drainage.

This morning I had a mini tarot reading with Sandra, another acquaintance. When I asked about my book I wasn't surprised to be told this was my way ahead. That morning I had asked for another name and Al Muqaddim came to me, which is to do with preparing for the way ahead. I am feeling much more positive about my future. I must find the emotion behind the fluid retention. I am beginning to sense it has to do with my emotional dependence on my children. As I have no partner, perhaps I have relied on them too much. I must let go now and learn to rely on my own strength, which I am learning I have. This was also indicated in the card reading.

THURSDAY 13th June

Went to the breast care centre yesterday to have more fluid drained away, apparently this is not uncommon and may have to be repeated several times, although they prefer the fluid to drain naturally. This can go on for several weeks. No one explained this to me which would have saved me stressing about it. On another level fluid retention is of course to do with emotions, unresolved emotional issues. In my case I believe it to be grief for the love I have never truly experienced in my life. On two separate occasions people have told me that my soul mate is in the world beyond this one and therefore I am destined to be alone. This is hard to accept. Is this is the final hurdle I need to overcome? Accepting that this is an experience which in this lifetime is not for me. Do I believe this? or it could be as I originally suspected, that I am becoming too emotionally attached to my family?

I should be going for an ECG today, but once again the Red Cross transport haven't been in contact. So boring to have to phone around waiting ages for a response. Such a waste of time and energy! In the end I had to cancel my appointment. I also cancelled my visit to London next week. This is because of the fluid situation. I also feel it's for the best, as I don't want to rely on the girls for emotional support. I miss them all so much. In fact I don't think I could have got through the treatment so far without their support. There are so many of us in a similar position. I suppose its an age thing. Perhaps one solution might be to try to do things here to support each other. I have a few ideas flying around my head but I need to get stronger first. I am aware that I have had a hell of a battering both physically and emotionally. Again, a week by the sea is what I crave for right now. Dream on. Its my brother's birthday today. Happy birthday Ian.

SATURDAY 15th June

Woke early today, 5am. I got up and made a cup of tea, builder's style, and why not. It can't hurt now and then. Generally I am feeling much better about everything. The hospital phoned regarding my appointment with my oncologist Dr. Graham. He still wants to see me next Tuesday in spite of my not having the ECG. So decisions will have to be made. Do I continue with any further treatment such as radiotherapy if this is offered, or do I go it alone from here? I feel it is done, finished, and as long as I continue to do the inner work and acknowledge all I have learnt through this experience all will be well. I must do some research and see what can be done to repair the slight damage to my heart caused by Herceptin, which is one of the chemo drugs.

I am also surprised to find myself feeling much more at home here in Glastonbury. Perhaps I am beginning to find my place here now. This could be because I have consciously made my mind up not to be so emotionally dependent on my family. Instead of being needy I am beginning to see their roles in my life in a different way. Fantastic. It is comforting to know there are so many of us in the same boat. At last, my confidence in myself is returning. I am feeling at peace and although my breast, or rather where my breast was, is still very sore, tight and numb I do feel stronger.

SUNDAY 16th June

Two thoughts were in my head as I woke this morning. I was ruminating about the talk I intend to give about my book and the following thoughts came to me. Firstly, the message of the rose and the fact that the rose carries both male and female sex organs means it is therefore perfectly balanced. For some, finding a partner and experiencing genuine love between two people brings balance. For others balancing the male and female aspects within the self will have the same result. Unity within self, so the key is balance, the one way to unity with the source, God, Love, however we choose to describe the Creator, the one source of all. Both ways require travelling inward through the heart. The road to enlightenment. Another thought that came to me was that through my journey with cancer I have learnt that I had reached a stage in myself where the only way forward is inwards, going more and more deeply into myself. The quote from the Sufi mystic Ibn Arabi confirms this: "to know thyself is to know your Lord." I have had to clear out all the emotional baggage that had caused the energetic blockages which eventually manifested in the physical; in my case, cancer. A part of me had to die to allow me to go deeper into who and what I am. This is what I now truly believe the journey has been about. Now I ask myself does this mean I can stop any further treatment, or am I looking for an excuse not to? I must be absolutely honest with myself.

The BUTTERFLY Journal

MONDAY 17th June

In my practice this morning I asked for a name to help with the healing of my heart, and surgery. I was given two names, Al Tawwab, meaning returning to rhythm, and Al Mumit, transition. Makes sense.

TUESDAY 18th June

It's my son's birthday today. Once again the transport didn't call last night so it was an anxious ringing round as soon as the office opened. It got sorted at the last minute. My meeting with Dr. Graham went much better than I thought it would. The lovely nurse Jane was there too. She had done the draining for me. Dr. Graham echoed the words of the surgeon, saying that the results were very good. After a short discussion. I surprised myself by agreeing to complete my treatment with a course of fifteen consecutive days of radiotherapy. I think this was because part of me wanted to finish what I had started, and secondly in fairness to the medical profession and their way of treating cancer to which I had agreed, and which I felt was the right thing to do. I begin my radiotherapy mid July. Five days a week for three weeks. Finally the fluid seems to be draining away of its own accord.

FRIDAY 21st June

It's the summer solstice so I expect all the New Agers will have been up the Tor, Glastonbury's famous landmark, this morning to celebrate. The swelling after surgery continues to reduce. I have very little pain, just a little numbness.

I had no idea how uncomfortable post-surgery could be. After I came round one of the nurses on the ward told me it would take about three weeks to recover. She must have been joking!! I am also getting sharp stabbing pains too, which are apparently to do with the nerve endings, and my fingers and feet continue to be numb. I am also feeling really cold, a side effect of chemo. The weather doesn't help: it is grey, cold, and rainy. I long for a sunny beach and the sound and smell of the sea. I decided to take the bus to Street, the next little town, only to discover my bus pass had expired. So I just went home. Happy days! Yesterday I wrote more on this journey so far. It feels good to have made a start.

SUNDAY 23rd June

I have taken note that I have been feeling a little under the weather these last few days I seem to be peeing more than usual. I am tired and felt a bit out of breath coming up the High Street after shopping, also a craving for sweet food which is of course is a huge no no. I am wondering if my blood sugars have been knocked out of sync. Yesterday a letter from my GP came asking me to make an appointment for my annual diabetic check up. Seventeen years ago, during a general medical MOT, my blood count was point one over what it should have been. I was told this meant I was classed as diabetic type two. I refused any medication and have managed it with diet ever since, so it will be interesting to see if this treatment has affected my blood sugar levels. It could be that I caught a chill waiting for the bus that I didn't take because of my expired bus pass, or that I had sat in the sun too long when the weather took a sudden turn for the better, going from one extreme to another. Whatever it was I don't feel good. I prayed asking for a name to help with my general health. I was surprised to be given the name Al Wali. This is to do with friendship. In order to make friends in the outer world we first need to make friends with all the inner aspects within ourselves. Inayat Khan comments that to be a friend is the essence of following in the footsteps of the Sufis, helping us to develop an interest in others. Beginning by tolerating and respecting ourselves, Samuel Lewis, another modern Sufi, tells us "sometimes it is easier to develop friendships with beings who are not physically present because they don't let us down. This includes angels and God. But this is a practice that is not without some danger." This was me to a T earlier in my life. After years of research I learnt how to avoid any danger. I describe this in detail in my book, The Way of the Rose.

TUESDAY 25th June

Woke to another mini revelation. The work I did in my clinic days is what I call Intuitive Diagnosis. A client would be sent to me with a physical or emotional problem which wasn't responding to any kind of treatment. Using my intuition and insight I was able to trace back through various life movements in the client's life to one or more situations, some often traumatic that had caused blockages in their energy body which eventually manifested as a physical disorder. Believe me this really can and does happen. Most of us are unaware of this. I could then sense a healing route to their recovery. I practised this work for over twenty six years, but I had never looked through my own time line (my description for this process). There was no need as I had enjoyed good health up to now. Also at that time I was not following in the footsteps of the Sufi masters and so was unaware of the 99 names or their use as remedies. Perhaps in the future I will be called back to this work and employ the use of the names as part of the healing process. Who knows. This by the way is what I have been describing as inner work. It is interesting that whilst I am rewriting my book The Way of the Rose I see so much tying in with the importance of the inner journey.

FRIDAY 27th June

My grand daughter has been staying with me since last Sunday. After she left I went to Wells with Caroline. Arriving home to an empty house I realised a huge part of my issues are that I no longer want to be alone. I thrive in community, in sharing. As a species we are not meant to live alone. Sadly so many of us are having to live alone these days. I suppose in the bigger picture there will be a reason for this?

Glastonbury is also a place where many of us are single. Interesting. To make matters worse I am a Gemini. I not only need my twin, but I need to communicate. Has the time come to address this and plan to do something about it. If so what can I do to rectify this?

MONDAY 1st July

The last couple of days my balance has gone again. I woke with it on Saturday. Its a bit like vertigo, so annoying. Today I have my appointment with the Radiotherapy Department. Perhaps this is why I am not feeling so good. Having gone through chemo and surgery and knowing the cancer has gone I now have to deal with probably more unnecessary invasion to my body. However I agreed at the start of this journey to see it through for reasons I have already explained. I have many questions regarding the radiotherapy treatment for whoever I see.

TUESDAY 2nd July

The appointment went much better than I had anticipated. I came away feeling much better about having the fifteen day course, which will begin on the 29th. Today I saw Gill, the lovely MacMillan nurse who has been so helpful. Gill told me she had a male client who saw one of the cards I had given her. It was of a blue butterfly. Apparently when he saw it he was moved to tears. Interesting, as I have called my account of this journey Butterfly. Gill gave him the card, which is exactly what I would have done.

All in all I am feeling well and positive. Mimi, my ex-sister in law, is coming to visit tomorrow and I am looking forward to seeing her.

WEDNESDAY 3rd July

The swelling is still slowly going down, although I am still numb, sore, and generally uncomfortable in the area where I had the surgery. Interesting that the cancer had manifested on my right side, our spiritual side. Dr. Jaffe says that cancer is a disease of the soul. Makes sense to me. If his assumption is correct am I having to be transformed so that my soul can complete its journey on earth in this lifetime? It saddens me to think people don't seem to realise the soul through needs as much healing as the physical body. Most of us are too concerned with the external life, feeding the ego, battling with other people's egos and desire for material gain. We need to learn humility. Stop being so competitive, greedy, self-centred and materialistic.

Another more detailed tarot reading with Sandra was very interesting. I wanted to compare her reading with the rune readings. The question in my mind as she spread the cards was what was behind the reason I had had to go through this journey with cancer? This was the response: the reason was to get me to do the necessary inner work to free myself of all the emotional baggage I had been carrying around since my childhood. This work will enable me to become balanced. Once this process is complete

I will be able to resume my work at a much deeper level. In the past I had had a tendency to take on too many projects, especially those taken on behalf of others. Time to put my own interests first. Stop being the pleaser. The whole journey has been to give me the opportunity to have a new beginning. I must take care not to backtrack. This includes social activities too. The cards indicated that I have the ability to draw the light out of the darkness within myself. It has occurred to me that when I have been in my darkest moments I have produced some of my best work. This shows me that another aspect of myself comes to the fore, and takes over to heal. This light comes through my art and writing, my creativity. It is a healing light. I still have some way to go before I am completely transformed. The new work will come through my book and paintings when I am ready. I have been told this many times before on different occasions, by different people. All of this has already been put in place by those in the higher realms of being who help us. Everything has been written already. All I need to do is allow my intuition to guide me I am now connected to Sophia, the divine feminine within myself. This is a gift which has come down through my matriarchal line. As this energy settles itself into my being I will gain strength and balance. Communication is an important part of my work to come. This will manifest through my book, which has the potential to be a success. There is definitely a move on the horizon again organized by other worldly helpers. No decision has been made yet as to whether I will move location. This will become more clear after September. All in all it looks a very bright and fruitful future. I hope so. Met Mimi off the coach, it was lovely to see her.

THURSDAY 4th July

I woke this morning after a very good night's sleep, with the following thoughts in my head: I must take my five year old child from my childhood garden and unite her with the divine feminine now within me. She must be a part of this too. We had both become separated from her energy. I did a little inner ceremony to bring about this balance. I was told it would be a three day process before the transition will be complete, starting tomorrow, but today is play day, and I am going to introduce Mimi to Glastonbury.

FRIDAY 5th July

We had a lovely day yesterday, good conversation, and healing through talking about our ex-husbands. Mimi and I had married identical twins!! A lot was put to rest. I began my inner work by meeting my inner child and taking her into my inner garden and into the presence of the divine feminine, which manifested as a brilliant white light so bright we couldn't see anything, but the air was scented with the most exquisite perfume of roses and there we wait for direction for the next step.

SATURDAY 6th July

The second day of the three day process – here is what happened: I woke with the sense that I needed to do my daily practice in my inner world, with my inner child. We went into a garden, the same one as yesterday and today we could see perfectly. We sat on a bench under a bower of roses. We chanted together. I heard the shrill sweet voice of my inner child chanting Al Karim – abundant expression. I was chanting Al Kahfid – diminishment, meaning when we feel a part of ourselves has diminished, been forgotten, or left behind. Al Kahfid restores us to wholeness. Perfect: my inner child now reunited with its grown up me can express itself fully, perhaps merging the gifts it was born with into the adult self. I noticed her zikhr (prayer) beads were made from tiny rosebuds. I also noticed a narrow stream running a few metres away from where we were sitting. I knew we had to lie in the clear sparkling water, reminding me of Jesus baptising people in the river Jordan. We lay there together in the cool stream as the water bubbled over us. As we lay there I had a strong feeling that all our ancestors from our matriarchal line were watching. I noticed my paternal grandmother was amongst them too. An echo of woman travelling back through time into nothingness.

I stayed for awhile in my inner garden before coming back in the day. Later I wandered down to the Town Hall where a Well Being Fayre was in process. I knew Teagan would be there and I felt I wanted to see her. She was there but I was drawn instead to a young Indian man called Kai, who was giving hand readings. I knew I needed this young man to read mine. His reading confirmed all that the runes, and cards had shown, but it also showed a healing was taking place with my inner child. The reading showed there was someone coming into my life to support me, and that my book would be successful. I asked if there was any indication of a move and he told me it would be irrelevant where I lived as it was the work to come that was important. It would be my choice whether I decide to relocate. He also told me this choice could not be made until I had healed myself from my past. He also indicated that I still had a connection with my ex-husband, but there was no indication that there was any work to be done on this issue. He said my hands told him I had a strong connection to the Sophia/Magdalene energy: the divine feminine energy within me was strong, showing the potential essence of who and what I am about, but as this energy has not fully integrated yet no decisions will or can be made until this process is complete. It is underway and provided I do the inner work should be completed by September. This information was also indicated in runes and tarot cards. All the time he was reading my hands I had a sense of Sheik Nazim, my teacher on my Sufi path, nodding and smiling. I am sure this was all arranged just to boost my confidence in my own intuition. Kai told me he also had a strong connection to the rose. Interesting. All three readings have basically told me the same thing, but the hand reading was much more detailed.

SUNDAY 7th July

I woke feeling really strong and excited for the future. I think I am beginning to see Glastonbury in a new light. I am more tolerant of the people, almost seeing them for the first time, finally feeling a part of the Glastonbury community. At last I am not fighting living here any more. I revisited my inner garden with my inner child and again did my zikhr. I felt the presence of Sheik Nazim, who led us both up three steps and into the energy of the divine feminine. I didn't see this as a personification, but just an energetic force. This energy enveloped myself and my inner child. The three of us embraced. My child was in front of me. I had my arms around her, my hands in front. When I looked at them I noticed I was holding two roses, a white one in my right hand, a red one in my left. As I put my hands together in a gesture of acknowledgement the two roses merged into one beautiful pink rose. Sheik Nazim put his hand on my head and prayed – a blessing, I thought. My head seemed to fill with a purple light. As I was returning to my room from my inner garden I sensed I had grown very tall and that hundreds of people had been watching the proceedings. I had a sense that my ex-husband had been there too. My inner child and I had been united. We were now as one. Sheik Nazim told me to go create a life and use my new connection to serve the good of the whole. I felt very blessed and humbled by the whole experience. This also showed me that our teachers are still able to guide us even from beyond the grave.

WEDNESDAY 10th July

Visiting my inner world this morning I found myself back in my garden again. My inner child was with me and I was watching her grow into a young woman, it was like having a twin. We merged into one and I knew the work was being completed. The same purple light shrouded me again, filling my entire being. I felt at peace. I sensed I was being told to stay quiet and be alone for the next three days. I intend to spend the time writing.

SUNDAY 14th July

I prayed for a name for the next phase of my journey. It is Al Batin, the hidden traveller. More inner work to do, which I know will ultimately have an effect on my life in the material world. It is also to do with preserving living wisdom until the time is right for it to find its place in the outer world. Biding time until the One decrees the time is right. I also sensed to chant Al Zahir, which is about working in the material world. combining the two will give me balance – the message of the rose. I am finding writing out my cancer journey a challenge, as it is revisiting memories I would rather forget, but reliving these memories is also healing as it puts them to rest so to speak.

MONDAY 15th July

I spent all day yesterday moving the furniture around in the flat, changing the energy, ending a chapter ready to enter a new one. Feels very good.

The BUTTERFLY Journal

WEDNESDAY 17th July

Today I have a treatment for my back. I know its gone out again. I was right, I needed quite a bit of work on my pelvis. Tomorrow I have my diabetic check up. It will be interesting to see if treatment has affected my blood sugar levels. I will get the results next week.

FRIDAY 19th July

Woke at 5am with sharp pains in my back. It really hurt when I breathed in. I made a cuppa and tried to read for a while. Its pouring with rain outside adding to my distress. It's also much cooler. Or of course it could be a reaction to the treatment. My head is flooded with information for my book, which is great. I had spent yesterday writing, making notes for 'Butterfly'. The printers phoned to tell me that there was a lot of interest in my book 'The Way of the Rose'. Went for a walk round the Abbey grounds, which helped with the pain. I think I must have slept awkwardly. Some of the incoming information is to make a rose essence to go with the book. Exciting stuff.

TUESDAY 23rd July

I should mention that I took Arnica after my surgery and I have massive bruising all over the area. It looked so bad I phoned a homeopath friend of Mel's to seek advice. I was told not to worry as it was a good sign, meaning the bruising was coming out. I was advised to bathe the area with rose water. She suggested that I delay the radiotherapy until the bruising has faded somewhat. The good news is that the numbness is going from my fingers and my right leg is less numb too. I am still feeling stiff after my back treatment, unfortunately I jarred it again on my way home. I asked for a name to help with the bruising, and received Al Khafid, meaning diminishment, helping with loss – my breast, hair and femininity.

WEDNESDAY 24th July

The bruising is still bad even though I am applying the rose water three times a day as instructed. Everyone is away, so I feel very much alone, no sense of belonging. Am I being prompted to go deeper inside myself? I went for a walk in the Abbey grounds, and I thought I sensed Sa'di, the 13th century Sufi who first introduced me to the path. This was the first time I had sensed his for many years. My thoughts turned to my daughters. Both have gone silent. I expect my youngest is preoccupied as she is pregnant again and my eldest daughter is dealing with her own health issues.

THURSDAY 25th July

In the outside world Boris Johnston has become Prime Minister!!! Interesting to observe that the media and those in the public eye are now using words like intuition when they probably don't have a clue as to what it really means. Perhaps this is an indication that people like myself need to speak out and try to explain. The good news is that finally the bruising is fading, it's turning yellow just as I was told it would. Hooray! I spent the afternoon writing, as it is too hot to be outside. Most unusual for the UK.

FRIDAY 26th July

Woke feeling down and lonely, but felt better after a phone call from my friend Magdalena in New York, it was so good to hear her voice. I cheered up. We reminisced about our time in Brighton. I miss the friends I made during my time there.

I had my results back from my diabetic check up. They were fantastic, all good, so the diet is working well. This cheered me up too, lifting my mood even higher. Later Blue Cedar phoned to let me know that the first print run of 'The Way of the Rose' was ready. Oh my God it's real. If only I didn't have this course of radiotherapy looming up. I think that's what was bringing me down, but I am determined to see it through. I guess its all to do with timing, which the runes had indicated, showing life would change in September.

SATURDAY 27th July

I am using the names Al Fatah, the opener and Al Mummit, the transformer. These names are to be recited throughout my treatment.

The bruising has faded a lot. I wish I knew what reaction to expect from the radiotherapy, because I just want to get on with the next chapter. Patience, and positivity. The feeling is definitely returning to my fingertips, but not my feet.

SUNDAY 28th July

I collected my books yesterday and I am delighted with them. I sold three straight away to a little book shop aptly called The Rose Garden, who also asked if I could produce some cards of the book cover design. Beth, the bookshop owner, also showed me some beautiful art work by a friend who passed last year, but whose work is being exhibited at the Magdalene chapel. Her work is a series of work in tribute to Mary Magdalene. I also called in at Glastonbury Galleries and saw an exhibition of art depicting the artist's impression of the divine feminine, with a particular interest in Mary Magdalene. Am I being told something here? She is popping up everywhere. 'The Way of the Rose' has a direct connection to the divine feminine too. I am bracing myself for the next three weeks of treatment.

MONDAY 29th July

First session of radiotherapy today. I started the day with my usual practice and the name Al Mummit came to me. It means transformation. In my mind I was amazed to find myself watching a butterfly emerging from a cocoon. The butterfly was blue, beautiful iridescent blue wings still damp unfolding as I watched. It didn't fly away, but just rested as if drying out its beautiful bright blue wings.

WEDNESDAY 31st July

I have endured three days of treatment now. Not a pleasant experience. Mostly because of being shut in a windowless darkened room and being pushed and pulled into place on a metal bed before the actual beam targets the selected area. The team of radiographers on the other hand are all so lovely it's forgivable and it's only for a few minutes once set up.

During my prayer time this morning I saw the cover for this account of my journey. It was not what I had in mind. I saw a sprig of white buddleia with a blue butterfly. Several other species of butterflies were hovering around the flower. The background was the blue of a clear summer sky. I was just wondering where I would find a white buddleia when the phone rang. It was Caroline. She was doing some gardening and invited me to join her for a tea break. When I arrived I couldn't believe what I saw. It was a white buddleia. She picked me a spray which I will photo or paint later. Synchronicity or what?

The Radiotherapy department is mostly run by a team of young men. It feels very strange lying half naked being pushed and pulled into position by these men young enough to be my grandsons, but as I have said they are very special, which takes away most of the embarrassment. I cannot fault them. I continue to bathe the area where my surgery was with rose water and I have now started to massage comfrey ointment to the area receiving the radiotherapy. My hair seems to be growing back well in spite of the fact it has always been slow to grow. I asked for a name to chant to help with the possibility of any side effects and received the name Al Jabbar, meaning repair, and restoration!

WEDNESDAY 7th August

Not much to report I am halfway through treatment and so far, so good. My book is selling really well – I have sold half the copies already and two shops here in town are stocking it. Both are on their second orders. My eldest daughter and youngest grand daughter are coming for a long weekend. I am looking forward to seeing them.

THURSDAY 8th August

Bad night's sleep. As no one phoned regarding tomorrow's transport this means yet again I will have to phone the office, a very tedious procedure as it takes ages to get through. This is all very stressful. I try to be laid back about it because I just want to get it over with, but if I miss an appointment it's added on at the end, so delaying the whole thing. However a driver called before I had time to call the office. Apparently he had been away and got back what he considered too late to phone me. I wish he had.

The BUTTERFLY Journal

FRIDAY 9th August

Another bad night This time caused by a bad dream, unnecessary to reveal the contents except to say it was about being frustrated with various situations. Last treatment this week and apparently a taxi is taking and returning me as there are no drivers available. I hope this means I won't have to make conversation on the journey. I was wrong, as both taxi drivers were very nice and used to stepping in for the Red Cross.

MONDAY 11th August

Had a lovely weekend with the girls even though I was too tired to do much. I expect it is the treatment. Just a few days left now. I am on the home straight, and then I will have done it. Amazing. I have decided I don't want any more treatments that may be offered, enough is enough.

WEDNESDAY 13th August

I am beginning to feel tired after treatment, although I am sure it is mostly to do with the stress of not knowing if a driver is going to turn up, and the daily two hour trips to Taunton and back. Still nearly done now. My throat is a little sore too, which apparently is normal. I am drinking gallons of rose water, which I know from my research can help heal the effects of radiotherapy. Tomorrow I have an appointment with Cardiology, then afterwards for an ECG. It will be interesting to see what that shows as I had refused the drug they offered me to rectify the heart problem; instead, I'm taking a tincture of rose, and hawthorn.

FRIDAY 16th August

D-Day! A long day yesterday as I had to wait a couple of hours after my last treatment for the appointment with the Cardiac team. I bought a little gift of appreciation for the boys in the Radiotherapy department. Just some extra-special biscuits. They have all been amazing. I caught up with Gill the MacMillan nurse, which was lovely and I promised her I would write my journey. The echo cardiogram wasn't too bad, I hope the results will be good. I was exhausted by the time I got back. How those medics work in those darkened rooms day after day I can't begin to imagine.

I am beginning to feel the need for some serious exercise. I just want to get back on form. Patience I guess. Although the bruising has significantly faded I am still finding even wearing a softie bra is very uncomfortable. Although I have had no significant side effects from the treatment I have been warned this can still happen a couple of weeks or even months later. So I will carry on drinking rose water, and massaging with comfrey ointment for at least another couple of weeks.

Well I am back from the last treatment and so finally its over – I've done it. It is a very strange feeling that after almost a year of treatment I am finally free. I feel very emotional about it. Several times today I could feel myself welling up, but for no apparent reason. Also I sense a little fear creeping in. Suddenly I am completely alone. I am on my own with the thoughts that it could return. Stay positive There is no reason why it should. Suddenly, after a year of a very close relationship with and support of my family, now I am out the other side so to speak, they have withdrawn. And why not, they have been absolutely amazing, but they all have their own lives too. It just feels very scary to be suddenly alone again. I now have to create a new life for myself. I asked for a name to help with this and was given Al Mu'izz – finding the stability and evidence of one's own beauty, grace, and the richness in ones own soul. High esteem! This enables one to find the confidence to manifest a new beginning, a new chapter which is absolutely the right direction. This feels very appropriate at the completion of this journey. Tomorrow will be the first day of the rest of my life. I must make sure I get it right. No one can possibly imagine what this journey has been like unless they have experienced it first hand. It really is a transformational life changing journey.

SATURDAY 17th August

After a very good night's sleep I woke feeling a sense of aloneness. It's all a bit of an anticlimax going from a year of treatment to suddenly nothing. In an almost perverse way I miss the thought of trips to the hospital, chatting to the Red Cross drivers and being treated so kindly by the medical teams. Plus the company of others going through the same ordeal, sharing understanding and in a strange way giving a sense of belonging, which I hadn't had in my life before my journey with cancer. Doesn't make sense does it? Well its up to me now to make something out of the rest of my life. I had a lovely message from the children telling me how proud they all are of me. It brought tears to my eyes. Their support played a huge part in getting me through this journey.

SUNDAY 18th August

Well its gradually sinking in, the end of the journey. I feel no surge of euphoria or jubilation. I don't know what I expected to feel, relief maybe at the least, but no, nothing. So now it's all about looking forward to a future. My book is finished and published, and so far it is being well received. I have the launch to look forward to and the talk for the Positive Living group, so lots to get on with. When I began this journey it was all about me having cancer, the physical disease that needed to be addressed and dealt with on the physical level, but I soon realised there was also much to sort out on an emotional and energetic level too. All previous life movements that had had an effect on my whole being had to be found and eliminated. I did this by going inward into my inner being and through my spiritual practice – in my case the use of the 99 names and prayer. There is no doubt in my mind that the strict diet at the beginning changed my mental attitude, giving me the positivity I needed to carry me through the harsh treatment I was about to face. The inner work gave me insight into all those times in my life that caused energy to stagnate, building to eventually manifesting in my case as cancer. It is so important we look within and empty out our rubbish so to speak. Some of the medical profession are beginning to recognize this concept which is great.

I believe working with the 99 names has played a major part in clearing and healing all aspects of my being and so preparing me for the future – truly a transformation. So my journey with cancer has taken me through a huge healing process in every aspect of my being. In a way I have to say thank you. I know that sounds mad, but it's what I feel. I am a very different person from the one I was at the start of this journey, and definitely for the better. I am now the butterfly ready to fly off into a warm sunny day and enjoy the beauty and perfume of the floral world.

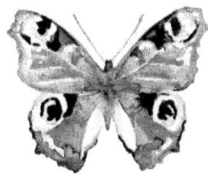

LIFE AFTER CANCER

Practicalities first: the following is a summary of everything that helped me through my journey with cancer.

Firstly, I took the time to get my head around what had happened to me. I didn't buy into all the fear mongering. I did my own research by looking at all options of treatment, being my own judge of what would be right for me and not allowing myself to be swayed by others, no matter how well their intentions were. Too many cooks so to speak. I did dither about at first. In order to be clear headed, I told no one except my three children and only one or two close friends. This was to safeguard me from becoming distracted. It made me stronger, although it still took a while before I really felt in control.

The gift box from my daughters containing Dr. T's PolyBalm for the nails, brilliant. Quease Ease for nausea which was fantastic. The lovely moisture balm for my sore nose (one of the side effect of the drugs), and a few luxury items such as two pairs of cashmere socks and some lovely cosy Ugg boots. The gift box idea is a must. Another effect of the chemo was I felt very cold, especially my hands and feet. No one had mentioned this might be a problem. So if someone you know is going through a cancer journey then a gift box is a lovely way to make their journey more bearable.

For me the diet was one of the most important decisions I made. I know it changed my mindset: Plant Paradox by Dr. Stephen Gundry was the book that was recommended to me. An alkali diet is one to follow, as well as taking all sugars out of the diet, even carbohydrates as they have sugar content too. No sweet fruits such as melons, bananas (unless under-ripe), mangoes and dried fruits. The best fruits to eat are berries. Research shows that cancer cannot survive in alkali conditions, and that tumours feed on sugar.

My daily writing of this journey has been invaluable, helping to release all the pent up emotions, fear and doubts. I would strongly advise anyone going through an ordeal such as cancer to do this. Spit them all out, don't swallow them and most importantly write them out. Writing can be a vital part of any healing process. I refer to this as inner work, which includes writing. By writing down my thoughts allows mental overthinking to relax. Sitting quietly and looking back through my life I saw what had made me angry. Did I feel unjustly treated by anyone? I looked at all the people who I felt had hurt me in some way. I had to be honest with myself. I had allowed those people to treat me in ways that were not acceptable. I forgave myself. I forgave them. I turned it round and looked at what had caused them to act in such a way. There was always a reason. I may have just been the trigger, but all these situations caused energy blocks in my physical body. These blocks need to be removed in order for all of us to enjoy a healthy and contented life. Its hard work but worth the effort. Once recognized and accepted it really does work. There are many ways to clear these energy blocks. Mine was by using the 99 names as I have described in this account, as well as my daily writing and the inner work through meditation and visualisation. Find a way that is right for you, a way you trust and believe in. Also, prayer is a very powerful tool, and coupled with sincerity of intention we can overcome even the most daunting challenges.

I hope my story illustrates that by working on every aspect of ourselves we can be instrumental in our own individual healing process. In fact, in order to make a complete recovery I believe it is essential. This is the holistic way to a healthy and happy life. We are not just flesh and blood. The body is simply the machine that contains all other aspects of being human. Just because we can't see them doesn't mean they are not just as an important part of us too. If everyone took this on board the world would be a much happier and healthier place. I see it like the pebble in the pond, the ripples could reach far and wide. Not observing this concept is just papering over the cracks. Also, we shouldn't dismiss the idea that there could just be an intangible force beyond human comprehension at work too. Readers will have observed that my own particular inner journey is following in the footsteps of the Sufis, which simply means following my heart and intuition to guide me through life. I had reached a point of my life where I had strayed from my path. My journey through cancer has not only led me back to my path but it has also given me the opportunity to clear out all that no longer serves me. At the end of my treatment I asked for a name; the name Al Muntaqim came to me. This name has a sweeping out and cleansing action, an appropriate name for the completion of this journey. Others will have their own paths. It doesn't matter which road you take as long as you have found one. The Brazilian writer Paoulo Coelho says, "God inscribed on the earth many paths, one for every man. It is just a question of finding the one that was written for you."

Readers might ask "How do I find my path?" The answer is simple. Pray, in whatever way you consider prayer to be, and pray with sincerity of intention: you only have to ask.

I appreciate that not everyone who reads this account of my journey will agree with me or even believe me, although I assure readers that this account is absolutely what happened to me on this transformational journey. My hope is that at least my story will give all those who read it some positive food for thought.

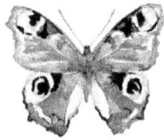

POSTSCRIPT

SUNDAY 6th October

I am sitting in the grounds of Glastonbury Abbey by the duck pond. It is a sunny day. The heat from the sun is strong. I have closed my eyes and when I open them I see that several dragonflies have settled themselves on my cardigan. I watch fascinated, their tiny iridescent bodies quivering in the rays of the sun. Heads turning this way and that, tiny wings, flashes of silver fluttering, indecisive as whether to take off again. Then when one took off they all flew away.

Back at home I have looked up the symbolism of the dragonfly which I knew, like the butterfly, was to do with transformation I found the following: Change – unmasking the real self and removing the doubts one casts on his or her sense of identity. Self discovery and removal of inhibitions. Change in the perspective of self realization. The kind of change that has its source in mental and emotional maturity and an understanding of a deeper meaning to life. The dragonfly's association with water represents the act of going beyond what is on the surface and looking into the deeper implications and aspects of life, giving support to making the necessary changes to be able to reach one's full potential.

Life is full of symbols, it is the language of the intuition. We just need to realise this. It is a free service provided by an intangible aspect of our life force. Some might consider this mystery to be God. Just because we can't see it at work doesn't mean it is not there guiding and supporting us always. This guidance is so subtle that it is so easy to miss it, but when we do it it can change our lives.

I am now engaged in an exciting new project. Me and two friends are organising a five day festival here in Glastonbury this summer, it's called the Rose Festival. The inspiration came after the success of my book 'The Way of the Rose'. The festival celebrates the uniqueness of this very special flower and the important message it carries for humanity which links in with so much with this account of my journey through cancer. The festival will include talks and demonstrations, an art exhibition and a concert. It is so good to be engaged in all aspects of life again.

Be well, go well: become you, and live.

Halima

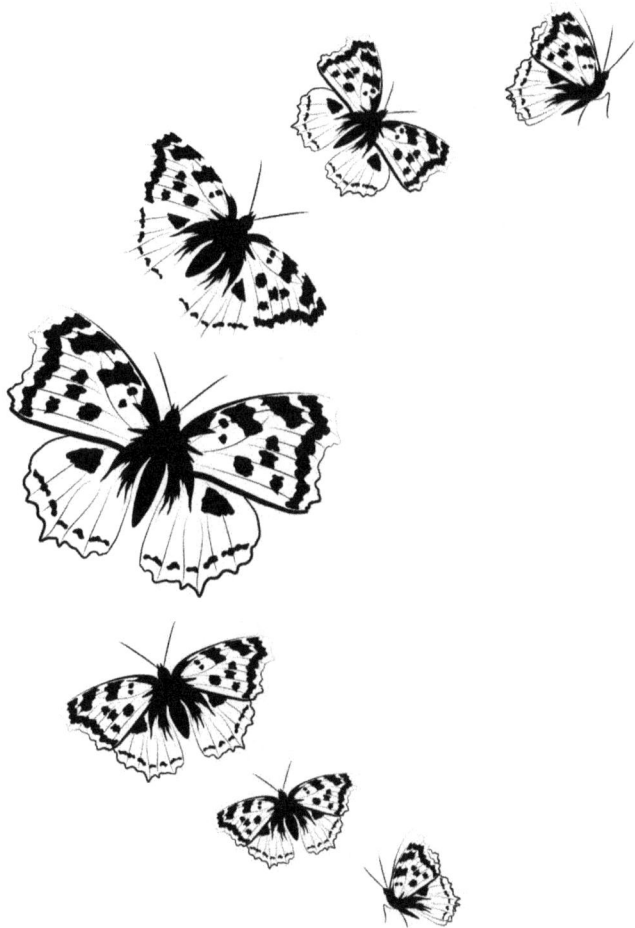

AFTERWORD

As a friend of Halima and having thirty years experience as a therapist myself, I have been overjoyed at the powerful inner work Halima has undertaken alongside chemotherapy and diet. By looking at, and altering, her mental and emotional state whilst receiving NHS support throughout the past year she has regained good health.

The practice of medicine has changed dramatically since the Egyptians used herbs and basic surgery around 3000 BC. The earliest known medical text book written in Sanskrit dates from approximately 600 BC. Hippocrates, the 'father of medicine' lived on Kos around 460 to 370 BC. As we move through Jenner's discovery of the smallpox vaccination in 1796 and on down the centuries, mankind has constantly searched for relief from pain.

Early wise men and women had an understanding of the relationship between cause and effect, taking into account their client's emotional and mental states during treatment.

More recently, allopathic medicine appears to have focused on incredible leaps in surgery and pharmaceutical remedies helping millions. However alongside that there has been a growing awareness of the need to treat the 'whole person'. So-called 'alternative' treatments are becoming mainstream. Many GPs practice acupuncture, refer patients for physio or to a chiropractor or osteopath. Some hospitals include such practitioners within their staff, along with counsellors and healers. Both Halima and myself have run clinics within hospitals.

For many people the idea of seeking help from anyone outside the NHS seems ridiculous, too expensive or downright scary, especially talking to a stranger about deeply personal issues. It can be very difficult to initiate change, be on a new diet, force oneself to take exercise, or admit to deeply hidden grief, guilt or anger. If one can do this, however, the relief and results can seem almost miraculous.

As we move on through the 21st century hopefully we will all become more and more aware of the inter-connectedness between our bodies, our state of mind and our suppressed emotions, leading us all to a healthier and more fulfilling life – there will be no more 'alternative' medicine as all disciplines will have their place.

Caroline, 2020

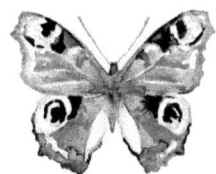